THE Nursing Clinics

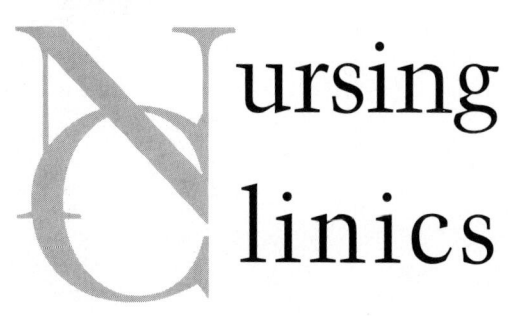

OF NORTH AMERICA

Nursing Problems of Persons with Cardiovascular Disorders

JOSEPHINE A. DOLAN, *Guest Editor*
Professor of Nursing, The University of Connecticut

The Nurse and the Ill Child

GLORIA LEIFER, *Guest Editor*
Department of Nursing Education,
City University of New York at Hunter College

MARCH, 1966

Volume 1, Number 1

W. B. SAUNDERS COMPANY, Philadelphia and London

© 1966 by W. B. Saunders Company. Copyright under the International Copyright Union. All rights reserved. This publication is protected by copyright. No part of it may be duplicated or reproduced in any manner without written permission of the publisher. Made in the United States of America. Press of W. B. Saunders Company.

The following information is published in accordance with the requirements of the United States Postal Code.

The Nursing Clinics of North America is published quarterly by W. B. Saunders Company, West Washington Square, Philadelphia, Pennsylvania 19105, at Hampton Road, Cherry Hill, New Jersey. Subscription price is $12.00 per year. Student subscription is $10.00 per year. Application to mail at second class postage rates is pending at Haddonfield, New Jersey.

This issue is Volume 1, Number 1.

The editor of this publication is Helen L. Dietz, W. B. Saunders Company, West Washington Square, Philadelphia, Pennsylvania 19105.

The following persons each own one per cent or more of the stock of W. B. Saunders Company: A. Paul Burton, John L. Dusseau, Harry R. Most, Sherman E. Perkins, Lawrence Saunders, Morton T. Saunders, W. Grier Saunders, T. Vanden Beemt, each of the W. B. Saunders Company, West Washington Square, Philadelphia, Pennsylvania 19105; Frances P. Kellogg, Emily S. Perkins, Dorothy L. Saunders, Sally L. Saunders, each of Bryn Mawr, Pennsylvania; Martha S. Ferguson, Swarthmore, Pennsylvania; Anna Holmes, Corning, New York; Margaret P. Manlove, Gladwyne, Pennsylvania; Charles C. Perkins, Jr., Atlanta, Georgia; and Nancy Gayle Saunders, Boston, Massachusetts.

Library of Congress catalog card number 66-17196.

Contributors

March, 1966

IMMACULATA M. ALBA, R.N., Hospital of St. Raphael, New Haven; B. S., New York University; M.A. in Medical-Surgical Nursing, New York University. Instructor, University of Connecticut School of Nursing. Instructor in Medical-Surgical Nursing and Educational Coordinator, Hospital of St. Raphael, New Haven, Connecticut.

IDA W. BALTIMORE, R.N., Fordham Hospital, New York; B.S. and M.A., New York University. Clinical Instructor, Fordham Hospital; Assistant Superintendent of Nurses, New York City Department of Hospitals at Metropolitan Hospital, New York

BARBARA M. BRODIE, R.N. and B.S., Loyola University, Chicago; M.S., Boston University. Assistant Professor of Pediatric Nursing, College of Nursing, University of Illinois, Chicago.

HELEN K. CHUAN, B.S., Winthrop College; M.N., Yale University. Instructor, University of Connecticut School of Nursing, Storrs, Connecticut.

JOSEPHINE A. DOLAN, R.N., B.S. and M.S., Boston University. Professor of Nursing, University of Connecticut School of Nursing, Storrs, Connecticut.

CLAIRE M. FAGIN, R.N., B.S., Wagner College; M.A., Teachers College, Columbia University; Ph.D., New York University. Assistant Professor and Director of Graduate Programs in Psychiatric-Mental Health Nursing, New York University School of Education, New York.

AUDREY J. FULCHER, R.N., Hartford Hospital; B.S., Boston University; M.A., Teachers College, Columbia University. Instructor, University of Connecticut School of Nursing, Storrs, Connecticut.

BARBARA M. GURSKI, R.N., St. Francis Hospital, Hartford; B.S., Boston College; M.A., Teachers College, Columbia University. Instructor, University of Connecticut School of Nursing, Storrs, Connecticut.

MARY JANE KENNEDY, R.N., St. Francis Hospital, Poughkeepsie, New York; B. S. in Nursing Education, Catholic University of America, Washington, D.C.; M. A., Fairfield University, Fairfield, Connecticut. Instructor, University of Connecticut School of Nursing, Storrs, Connecticut.

CONTRIBUTORS

GLORIA LEIFER, R.N., Fordham Hospital School of Nursing, New York; B.S., Hunter College, New York; M.A., Teachers College, Columbia University. Lecturer in Maternal-Child Nursing, Department of Nursing Education, City University of New York at Hunter College, New York.

KAREN H. McARDLE, R.N., St. Therese Hospital, Waukegan, Illinois; B.S., Teachers College, Columbia University. Instructor, Misericordia Hospital School of Nursing, Bronx, New York

EUGENIA C. MOTOCK, R.N., Michael Reese Hospital, Chicago; B.S. and M.A., Ohio State University. Assistant Professor, University of Connecticut School of Nursing, Storrs, Connecticut.

JANICE PAPEIKA, Senior Student, University of Connecticut School of Nursing, Storrs, Connecticut

ELEANOR RUDICK, R.N., Newark City Hospital; B.S. in Education, Hunter College; M.A. and Ed.D., Teachers College, Columbia University. Assistant Professor, Department of Nursing Education, Teachers College, Columbia University, New York.

DORSEY IVEY SMITH, R.N. and B.S., Duke University: M.A.; Teachers College, Columbia University. Instructor in Obstetric Nursing, Cornell University-New York Hospital School of Nursing, New York.

SHIRLEY STEELE, R.N., Waterbury Hospital; B.S. in Nursing Education, M.A. in Maternal and Child Health Nursing, Teachers College, Columbia University. Public Health Nursing Consultant, Children's Rehabilitation Center, Buffalo; Part Time Assistant Professor of Public Health Nursing, State University of New York at Buffalo.

PAULINE F. TEPE, B.A., Mount Mercy College, Pittsburgh; M.S. in Zoology, Marquette University; M.N., Frances Payne Bolton School of Nursing, Western Reserve University. Graduate Teaching Assistant in Human Anatomy, University of Arizona, Tucson.

MARY JANE VENGER, R.N., Presbyterian Hospital, Pittsburgh; B.S., University of Pittsburgh; M.A. in Nursing Science Administration, Teachers College, Columbia University. Director of Nursing, Mount Sinai Hospital, New York.

HELEN T. WATSON, R.N. and B.S., University of Connecticut; M.S., Yale University. Assistant Professor, University of Connecticut School of Nursing, Storrs, Connecticut.

HARRIETT L. WILCOXSON, R.N. and B.N., Yale University; M.A., Teachers College, Columbia University. Assistant Professor of Public Health Nursing, University of Connecticut School of Nursing, Storrs, Connecticut.

Contents

SYMPOSIUM ON NURSING PROBLEMS OF PERSONS WITH CARDIOVASCULAR DISORDERS

Foreword 1
    Josephine A. Dolan, Guest Editor

Coping with Emotional Stress in the Patient
Awaiting Heart Surgery 3
    Mary Jane Kennedy

A Patient with Sarcoma of the Pericardium 15
    Eugenia C. Motock

Rationale of Nursing Care for Patients with
Blood Dyscrasias 23
    Barbara M. Gurski

The Role of the School Nurse in the Support of
Children with Certain Cardiovascular Disorders 31
    Helen T. Watson

Impaired Pulmonary Circulation Due to
Pulmonary Emphysema 39
    Helen Chuan

The Nurse and the Patient with Peripheral
Vascular Disease 47
    Audrey J. Fulcher

The Nurse's Role in Preventing Circulatory
  Complications in the Patient with a Fractured Hip 57
    Immaculata M. Alba and *Janice Papeika*

Cerebrovascular Accident: The Role of the
  Public Health Nurse 63
    Harriett L. Wilcoxson

SYMPOSIUM ON THE NURSE AND THE ILL CHILD

Foreword 73
    Gloria Leifer, Guest Editor

Nursing and the New Pediatrics 75
    Eleanor Rudick

Pediatric Rooming-In: Its Meaning for the Nurse 83
    Claire Fagin

The Nurse's Reaction to the Ill Child 95
    Barbara Brodie

Administrative Responsibilities of the Pediatric Nurse 103
    Ida Baltimore

A Physiological Approach to Pediatric Medications 111
    Pauline Tepe

The Nurse's Role in Fetal Medicine 121
    Dorsey Ivey Smith

Hyperbaric Oxygenation: Nursing Responsibility in Planning
  for a New Clinical Service 131
    Mary Jane Venger

The Patient and the Bennett 143
    Karen H. McArdle

The Role of the Public Health Nurse in the Discharge
of the Handicapped Child to the Community 153
    Shirley Steele

SPECIAL FEATURES

An Eminent Personality in Nursing:
  Lucile Petry Leone 165

A Problem in Interpersonal Relations:
  Telling the Truth to Leukemic Children 167

The Way It Was:
  Leeching 170

FORTHCOMING SYMPOSIA

June, 1966

INTERPERSONAL RELATIONS
Luther Christman, R.N., Ph.D., *Guest Editor*

INJECTION THERAPY: THE NURSE'S RESPONSIBILITIES
Anna L. Seal, R.N., *Guest Editor*

September, 1966

CHRONIC DISEASE AND REHABILITATION
June S. Rothberg, R.N., Ph.D., *Guest Editor*

December, 1966

THE NURSE AND THE NEW MACHINERY
Ruby M. Harris, R.N., M.S., *Guest Editor*

MENTAL RETARDATION
Kathryn Barnard, R.N., Ph.D., *Guest Editor*

Symposium on Nursing Problems of Persons with Cardiovascular Disorders

FOREWORD

Professional nursing has a unique role in health care, an abiding interest in humanity, and the ability to assist in promoting human welfare, preventing illness and caring for the sick patient. In this age of the explosion of knowledge and of scientific advances permeating all aspects of our dynamic culture, the basic needs of man continue to blaze forth as the chief and primary concern of nursing. But at this point in time the principles of scientific research must be used by nurses in the solution of the health problems of man.

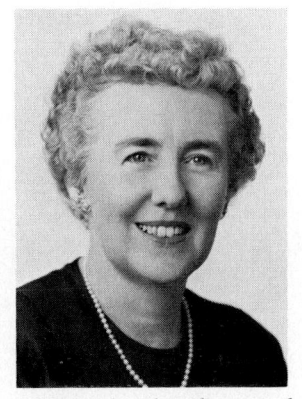

Professional nurses are challenged to assist individuals, families, and communities in achieving optimum levels of well-being. The desirable level to be achieved by each individual needs study and delineation. Clinical practice is the focus and heart of nursing and it is through the practice of nursing that we fulfill our obligation to society.

The authors of the following series of articles felt that the nature and magnitude of one of the nation's major health problems, that of disturbances of circulation, merited attention. They were concerned by the staggering loss of economic productivity due to disability and premature death, and by the trauma to the patient and his family, which faces suffering, loss of human dignity, and disruption of the family unit.

In the following papers the supportive role of the nurse is shown principally through a series of case studies. The professional practice reported on took place in hospitals, homes, and schools. In each setting the practitioner becomes involved in a myriad of functions related to her role of providing care for the person with a circulatory disturbance. She may be called upon to provide emotional support, as for the patient awaiting open heart surgery and for the person with a fatal illness such as sarcoma of the pericardium. She may function as an educator, as with children with cardiovascular disorders or patients with peripheral vascular disease. She may help in the rehabilitation of the victim of a cerebrovascular accident. In every instance, however, the nurse performs her role in the promotion of human welfare and in meeting the basic needs of her patients.

JOSEPHINE A. DOLAN
University of Connecticut
School of Nursing

Coping with Emotional Stress in the Patient Awaiting Heart Surgery

by MARY JANE KENNEDY, M.A.*

In 1948 Dr. Charles Bailey of Philadelphia and Dr. Dwight Harken of Boston both began to employ at about the same time the procedure of direct digital approach to the heart. As a result of that remarkable event, we in nursing have experienced the challenge and the privilege of caring for the cardiac surgical patient. It has been approximately ten years since cardiac surgery became feasible in the general hospital, and as we look back on the excitement of those first years, we recall our initial reactions. How amazed we were at the scientific and technologic progress which permitted the beating heart to be invaded! How proud we were of the skill of our cardiac surgeon! How much we admired those fantastically courageous pioneer patients!

Because of the long period of preoperative evaluation and preparation there developed, between nurse and patient, a special relationship, as we helped him with his physical care, prepared him for a myriad of laboratory tests, and guarded him against any complication that might result in postponement of surgery. As a result of this close relationship we became conscious of the patient's fear, and as the day of surgery drew near, we spent as much time with him as possible, realizing what our presence meant in this period of stress. On the operative day, the hospital "grapevine" carried periodic bulletins of the progress of surgery. The patient had "made it" so far. All was well! We heaved a sigh of relief for the surgeon, for the hospital, but above all for our patient whom we could hardly wait to see again.

---

* Instructor, University of Connecticut School of Nursing, Storrs.

TRENDS IN CARDIOVASCULAR NURSING CARE: PRIORITY OF INTEREST

In the ensuing years, we seem to have become quite sophisticated about cardiac surgery. The patient who is a candidate for a procedure on the mitral valve is no longer a novelty, and we regard a closed valvulotomy as being almost as routine an operation as any other major surgery. Meanwhile, we are witnessing even greater achievements in this field. The heart is being stilled. Terms like "cardiopulmonary bypass," "hypothermia," "monitor," "pacemaker" and "prosthetic valve" are part of our everyday vocabulary. Higher risk patients with multiple cardiac defects are being brought to surgery, and the complex and complicated problems of postoperative "intensive care" have caught our attention, as can readily be seen by the generous amount of interesting and valuable literature available on the subject. This priority of interest in postoperative care is reflected, too, in the activity of the surgical patient care areas, where the attention is preeminently focused on the patient with the "beeping" monitor and the bubbling chest tube.

As a result of the increasing complexity of cardiovascular surgery, groups of highly specialized personnel have emerged who form a "cardiac team" or "pump team," with esoteric functions and responsibilities related to the patient's management before, during and immediately after surgery. To this group might be added the intensive care nursing team, who are located in a special area, usually apart from the unit or division where the patient resides preoperatively. One wonders if this inevitable specialization of function and fragmentation of responsibility for the care of these patients, along with the higher priority of interest in postoperative nursing care, has not created a lessening of responsibility and a casualness on our part toward the candidate for cardiac surgery. Are we, who still have the responsibility for preparing these patients for surgery, losing sight of our place in the schema? Or are we simply forgetting a fact of which we were most keenly aware ten years ago—that these patients are extremely frightened, and that, as yet, there is no special team designed to help them cope with their stress.

THE PREOPERATIVE PERIOD—THE "COUNT DOWN"

How does the patient spend his time preoperatively? Even though the use of preliminary services on an outpatient basis has shortened this period somewhat, we find that the admission date for the average candidate for open heart surgery is seven to ten days prior to the procedure. During this time the patient is usually placed in a single room in order to minimize the hazard of upper respiratory infection, to which he is generally highly susceptible. Restrictions are even more rigid in some medical centers. All personnel and visitors must don a mask as they enter the room, or else must stand outside the doorway. Young children of the candidate may not visit. When the patient leaves his room, he, too, must wear a mask.

What do these restrictions mean to him? How do they affect the family and visitors? No doubt the patient knows the importance of protection, but the seriousness of the impending procedure may be magnified by the rituals of isolation. Are we concerning ourselves with this possibility? To whom do the patient and family turn for understanding at this time?

As the days drag on, the candidate for open heart surgery finds himself with an increasing amount of time on his hands. Last minute tests are complete and, barring complications, he and his family await the scheduled day. If he is fortunate, he meets a convalescing heart surgery patient down the hall, or another preoperative patient or family member with whom he can commiserate. Candidates for heart surgery seek to reduce their anxiety through identification with one another, which can be a healthy experience. Occasionally, however, erroneous comparisons are made or misinformation is acquired, of which the nursing staff is often unaware. Occasionally, too, the preoperative patient becomes very apprehensive when he sees that a fellow heart patient, on return to his room after surgery, is attached to a device—a monitor that triggers constantly. Are we concerning ourselves with the impact of these occurrences on him? Or do we count on the patient's television set to keep him from worrying? The fact that is most disquieting is that, too often, the other patients know the candidate for cardiac surgery and his fears better than do the nurses.

It is well past time to ask ourselves these questions. How often do we dash in and out of the patient's room "armed" with a syringe, a stethoscope, or a specimen container? Or how often do we plan a time to spend in conversation with him, not just intuitively, but with the realization that a patient about to undergo heart surgery is experiencing extreme stress regardless of his overt behavior? How prepared are we to identify the mechanisms used by our patient to cope with his stress, some of which may have a very undesirable effect postoperatively? Why aren't we preparing ourselves to better understand the preoperative patient as eagerly as we seem to want to learn how to read monitors, to operate pacemakers, and to trigger positive pressure machines?

UNDERSTANDING STRESS

The phenomenon of stress—its origin, manifestations, and effects—is, of course, largely within the domain of psychology and psychiatry. Principles determined by the results of research and investigation in these areas, however, have broad implications for all members of the health professions.

One of the most comprehensive and interesting references for those engaged in health services is *Psychological Stress* by Professor Irving Janis of the Department of Psychology at Yale University.[1] Using surgery as a stressful experience, Dr. Janis presents a psychoanalytic study of a patient who underwent a surgical procedure during a period of psychotherapy. He also intensively studied approximately 30 patients before and after surgery in order to analyze the behavioral changes that occurred as a result of their total experience. He analyzed the data from these case histories, and from a questionnaire covering over 200 male adolescents who reported their reactions to both major and minor surgery, and developed a set of hypotheses, the last three of which are germane to this discussion because they are concerned with a display of preoperative fear. Dr. Janis grouped his patients according to an estimate of degree to which "anticipatory fear" was displayed (high, moderate, and low). He determined that those who display—or who are given an opportunity to display—moderate fear will be less likely to suffer emotional disturbance after the experience than those who display either a high or a low degree of fear. He characterized the group having high anticipatory fear as being likely to continue to demonstrate fear of bodily damage after the threat of surgery has passed. The patients with low anticipatory fear, according to Dr. Janis, are more apt to be angry and resentful of what he calls "danger control authorities"—doctors and nurses—after the crisis period.

Applications to Nursing. Although Dr. Janis' hypotheses are obviously intended to be utilized by psychiatrists and psychologists in counseling surgical patients, he makes many applications of his theories which could be useful to other members of the health professions. A broadening of our own background may well open our eyes to the signals being given by an anxious preoperative patient. How do we handle questions that are posed to us about the surgical procedure? Or are no questions asked of us? We are usually cognizant of the need for the very apprehensive patient to receive help, but what about the so-called "well adjusted" patient who appears to display little or no anticipatory fear?

Dr. Janis declares that some of the most severe postoperative stress is experienced by this individual who appears to have little or no preoperative fear, because he has not beforehand been able to develop anxiety-reducing defenses that usually accompany "worry," and that serve as coping mechanisms once the danger situation has arrived. When we observe that a patient does not wish to be informed about the experiences that he is about to undergo, or that he cannot bring himself to discuss any aspect of the surgery, to whom do we transmit this information? What is our plan of care for the candidate who becomes aware of the death of a postoperative "open heart" patient?

How do we use what we know about the behavior of people under stress in planning nursing care? For example, we know from the study of psychology that the senses of people under stress are not efficient. What is heard or seen is not always perceived correctly and is easily forgotten. When a patient's orientation is planned, therefore, to such experiences as the recovery room, the postoperative exercises, the pain, and the positive pressure respirator, how do we evaluate the integration of this information? Do we automatically assume that the physician has made all this stressful information abundantly clear? Conversely, do we condemn others for preparing the patient poorly when he seems unaware of what lies ahead? Perhaps this patient has not been able to assimilate all the data, and what we should be criticizing instead is our own lack of appreciation of what happens when infomation is given to people under stress. It is difficult to defend the position that we are individualizing our nursing care when we characterize patient after patient as "cooperative and cheerful" in our observation notes. Do they really all fit into the same benign behavioral mold? Or are we merely giving evidence of the fact that we do not really know this person who is a patient?

THE PATIENT'S REACTION TO HIS PREOPERATIVE CARE

How does the patient regard the nurse in the preoperative period? In seeking answers, this writer interviewed three convalescing patients with whom she had contact pre-less and postoperatively, while giving clinical instruction and supervision in cardiovascular nursing. Each person was chosen because of factors that would presumably heighten the stress of the operative experience: namely (1) the return of symptoms after a previous heart operation, necessitating reoperation, and (2) postponement of the scheduled procedure, necessitating readmission and/or a prolonged preoperative period. The writer asked each interviewee to recall only the events and the staff nursing personnel he or she encountered in the preoperative period (all three had private duty nursing care postoperatively). The purpose of this paper was not revealed until all questions were answered.

The questions that were posed to the interviewees were worded, in general, according to the following categories:

1. What experiences in the preoperative period bothered you the most?

2. What kind of help did you expect of the professional nursing personnel in the preoperative period to meet these distresses? Did the help you received meet your expectations of the help you sought?

3. Did you think the nurse played a significant part in your preoperative period?

4. Did you feel like talking to the nurse about your impending surgery? If so, what time of the day did you most feel like talking to her? From which group of nurses (day-evening-night) did you feel *least* removed; *most* removed?

5. How well do you feel you were prepared for the surgery by your nurses?

6. Did you see any difference in the kind of care you received preoperatively from the R.N., the L.P.N. or the aide?

7. Did you tend to seek out other cardiac patients, on the division, as diversion or for companionship?

Interview No. 1.   Mrs. F.—A Patient Who Underwent Previous Heart Surgery

The first interviewee was a housewife and mother of four, who had successfully undergone insertion of a "caged ball" prosthetic mitral valve 17 months prior to the interview. She had experienced a closed valvulotomy four years previously, but in the interval experienced a return of symptoms: progressive fatigue, shortness of breath, fluid in the lungs, and palpitations. Mrs. F. is an inactive professional nurse and had made it abundantly clear during her hospital stay that she wished to be regarded as a layman during this operative experience. During the interview she stated that she emphasized this point because she "did not wish to be given preferential treatment," although she also admitted that she was afraid that the staff would suspect her of being a "know-it-all."

Mrs. F. revealed that she was most distressed by her fear of impending death; in her own words "I knew I was slipping." She also recalled being distressed about the number of times her case had been presented for a decision about surgery, only to be put off because she was "not ripe." Between her first and second heart operations, she had a total of six admissions for return of symptoms.

Mrs. F. outlined her expectations of the nurse as the person responsible for (1) giving medications, (2) monitoring vital signs,

(3) preparing patients for laboratory studies, and (4) giving physical care as required. Since her nurses engaged in these activities, Mrs. F. felt that her expectations of the nurse's role were met.

In response to whether or not nursing played a significant role in her preoperative period, Mrs. F. became ambivalent toward her "sisters" in the profession. While excusing them as being too busy to accomplish more than what was outlined above ("it's a hectic profession"), Mrs. F. admitted that she did not think the nurses played a significant role at this time because of "a lack of close contact" with her as a patient. She sought specific information about the surgery from the doctors only, because she felt they would tell her "only what she should know," although she admitted that it was difficult to wait for the surgeon to answer her questions because she saw him so infrequently. She did feel, however, that she appreciated most talking with the evening nurses when she was alone "after the company went home." She rated her evening nurses as the ones from whom she felt *least* removed, and the day and night nurses equally as the ones from whom she felt *most* removed.

In answering question No. 5, Mrs. F. felt that she was not prepared by the nurses for the experiences of the immediate postoperative period. There were many areas, she said in retrospect, for which she would have wished preparation (i.e., recovery room experiences: hypothermia, the monitoring devices, the numerous "I.V.'s", and the intermittent positive pressure therapy).

In response to question No. 6, Mrs. F. saw little differentiation in the care she received from R.N.'s, L.P.N.'s, or aides. "Everyone was wonderful to me. They couldn't do enough for me" (enough was defined as the four items mentioned before).

At the termination of the interview, Mrs. F. stated that she thought the nurses could play a "tremendous role" in the preoperative preparation of a patient "but they don't have the time."

Interview No. 2. Miss M.—A Patient Whose Surgery Was Twice Canceled

Miss A.M. is a young psychiatric social worker with a history of chorea since age 14 who entered the hospital for a valvulotomy under the closed technique. Miss M. had been experiencing dyspnea on exertion for approximately four months prior to admission, and had sustained but recovered from an embolic episode affecting her left side approximately three weeks prior to admission. She was admitted February 22 of the current year and discharged three days later for the week-end because of operating schedule difficulties. On readmission, her prothrombin time was persistently low, and the operation was again postponed until March 5 at which time Miss M. underwent successful commissurotomy, followed by an uneventful recovery period.

The writer interviewed this patient approximately four months after surgery. Again, the same set of questions were posed. Miss M. revealed that she was, of course, most distressed by the postponement of her surgery—angered in fact, by the first postponement—and reentered the hospital in a somewhat unhappy frame of mind. To add to her distress, she discovered on readmission that some "used equipment" from a previously discharged patient had not been removed from her room. She had recalled, from her first admission, that this patient had been on isolation postoperatively for what she presumed to be a "staph" infection, so that the sight of this equipment "frightened and infuriated" her. According to Miss M. she received no help from the nurses with her problems. She reiterated her concern about the equipment for several days before it was removed.

Miss M. was an avid reader and enjoyed watching television; therefore, she was content to be located in a single room. She did not seek the companionship of other cardiac surgical patients until a physician recommended that she visit one such convalescing patient. Miss M. stated that most of the patients awaiting open heart surgery were "very frightened," and since she had made her mental preparation beforehand, she chose not to seek them out lest they begin to frighten her.

Miss M.'s expectations of nursing's part in her preoperative period were not met. She stated, for example, that she anticipated the head nurse would stop in to introduce herself, and she expected some structured orientation to the hospital and to the experiences she was about to undergo; in her own words "I expected the R.N. to greet me, ask me why I am here, and help me to be reassured." Her expectations did not materialize to any degree. When asked why she expected these approaches from the nursing staff, she replied that such an orientation was given to patients admitted to the hospital where she worked "and because I didn't get it on my first admission." When the surgery was postponed the second time, Miss M. stated she expected sympathetic reassurance from the nurses, but recalled that the only person who stopped by to comfort her was a nurse's aide.

In answer to question No. 3, Miss M. flatly summarized her negative feelings about preoperative nursing care by indicating that the R.N. was of no significance to her whatsoever, other than as "a dispenser of pills." She said she felt most removed from the R.N.'s and felt closest to a licensed practical nurse on evening duty, who took the time to stop by her room and chat briefly each day. Miss M. indicated that her greatest need for companionship and solace occurred between 3 p.m. and the dinner hour.

This interviewee admitted that her negative feeling toward nursing was undoubtedly colored by the postponements of her surgery, especially the initial one. Even now she looks upon this postponement as causing the greatest amount of stress for her, because it was an occurrence for which she was not at all prepared. She feels, however, that her expectations of nurses' functions were in no way met, and stated to this writer that she "often wondered how other patients ever managed postoperatively without private duty nursing care."

Interview No. 3. Mr. T.—A Patient Who Was Preoperative for 19 Days

The final interview was conducted with a 54-year-old patient who successfully underwent replacement of both the mitral and aortic valves with "caged ball" prostheses—a procedure which carries with it a rather high risk at present. Although Mr. T. sustained a heart block postoperatively, he is being very satisfactorily maintained with the aid of a radio frequency pacemaker. The interview was conducted five months after surgery.

Mr. T. is no stranger to life-threatening experiences, which was obvious at the hospital and at the time of interview. An ex-racing car champion and ex-pilot, he has had severe heart disease "for years." Mr. T. was "not afraid to die." He was, in fact, "looking forward to the surgery" without which, he had been warned, he "would not survive the summer." Mr. T. has little patience with signs of weakness. He often stated, during the interview, "I don't whine—I can't stand whiners."

Mr. T. answered all the questions in a general fashion He claimed to have little or no preoperative distress, although his surgery, too, was postponed. (He was admitted March 4 to have surgery March 11 but this was postponed until March 23 and he remained as an inpatient for this interval.) He admitted, later, to having been very disappointed but not upset when the scheduled surgery was postponed. A heavy smoker, Mr. T. failed to cut down adequately, and for reasons related to his pulmonary status operation was postponed until March 23.

Mr T. claimed he had a most satisfactory preoperative period. "I really wasn't sick so there were no problems," he said. During this time, he saw the nurses as persons who were "overworked," who "were too busy to talk to you," and "who had no time to pass the time of day with you." Like Mrs. F., Mr. T. felt that he had expected nothing other than physical care from the nurses; therefore his expectations were met. Mr. T. had experienced a great deal of support from his local physician, and had been given, according to himself, thorough preparation by the cardiac surgeon preoperatively. He saw no difference in the care he received from R.N.'s, L.P.N.'s, or aides except that he thought that the L.P.N.'s gave "more care" while the R.N.'s "gave medications."

Mr. T. accepted postponement of surgery until March 23 without question. He continued to smoke, when not supervised. He became friendly with all the patients on the division, including the cardiac patients, and concurred with Miss M.'s comment that the other cardiac preoperative patients "were frightened to death, but not me." He avoided lengthy conversation about heart surgery with other patients, saying "I don't listen to laymen." He did not discuss his impending procedure with his nurses because he "did not think the nurses knew that much about the procedure." In retrospect he feels that he was least prepared for the recovery room period (which he "hated"), although he had been given specific instructions about the activities that took place there. In general, he saw the nurses as hard-working people who had "no time for you" because there were "sick" patients on the unit "and I wasn't sick."

It is interesting to note that this writer's choice of interviewees resulted in views of an essentially similar nature about the nurse, as seen by three patients, two of whom one might call sympathetic toward nursing, and one of whom was not sympathetic.

CONCLUSIONS: HOW CAN WE BE MORE EFFECTIVE?

Although these interview summaries are offered for discussion purposes only, they bear out some of the criticisms that we nurses have already heard from both within and outside the profession. It would seem that the public expects little more than sympathetic, willing ministrations of a technical nature from those undifferentiated persons whom they regard as nurses. They do not regard us as playing a significant role in their preoperative care, and look to others—even other patients—for assistance in the area of emotional support and anxiety reduction. They charitably excuse us on the basis of our being too busy to meet more than their physical needs.

To comfort ourselves on this same basis—to be satisfied with this level of functioning—while at the same time to expect to be awarded professional status is inexcusable.

From the observations of this writer, it is a distressing but undeniable fact that a preoperative heart surgery patient is usually regarded as requiring, if not deserving, a minimal amount of nursing care.

Because he is "up and about" he is often assigned to the member of the nursing staff who is least knowledgeable, by standards of educational preparation, in the area of understanding human behavior. The alternative seems to be one of giving him to a staff nurse with an already overloaded assignment "because he only needs to have his bed made." How often has this writer been asked, when assigning a student to such a person, if she really wouldn't prefer a "more challenging" patient for her senior student! It can only be assumed that the rationale for taking such a position is either our limited appreciation of the impact of the stressful experience of awaiting open heart surgery *and its challenge,* or our own conviction that helping a patient to cope with his stress lies entirely outside of the domain of nursing.

Although the reaction to both these assumptions will be one of indignant denial, the facts speak for themselves. But need this be the case? If lack of time is the answer, the argument lacks substance. The time would be found for this same person were he a fresh postoperative patient. Is it lack of know-how? Let us, then, become better prepared so that we can devise a plan of care based on an awareness that the stress of this patient may not be as easily monitored as his damaged mitral valve, but is just as real. Then let us use the knowledge we have gained about the mechanisms of stress to alter the situation and equalize the focus of interest in the care of the cardiovascular patient. Assign this patient to the nurse who is most knowledgeable about the dynamics of behavior—let her have enough time to interview the patient, to exchange information, and to evaluate his reaction to the impending procedure. Give the patient information only as he can assimilate it, and discuss in staff conference his coping behavior.

Lastly, let us remember not only that fear is a natural phenomenon of the preoperative period, but also that this patient should be given opportunity to work out his worry with a truly observing, professional nurse close at hand to pick up clues that may indicate a need for further help.

REFERENCES

1. Janis, I. L.: Psychological Stress. New York, John Wiley and Sons, Inc., 1948.
2. Chodoff, Paul, Friedman, S. B., and Hamburg, D. A.: Stress, defenses, and coping behavior. Am. J. Psychiatry, 120:743–749, 1964.
3. Marshall, S. L.: Communication under stress. Internat. Psychiatric Clinics, 1:247–261, 1964.

73 Edgewood Avenue
New Haven, Connecticut 06511

A Patient with Sarcoma of the Pericardium

A Case Study

by EUGENIA C. MOTOCK, M.A.*

Malignant tumors of the pericardium remain one of the most difficult problems confronting medicine today. Laboratories throughout the country are constantly working on methods of preventing or curing this condition, but as yet no entirely satisfactory solution has been found.

The impact of crisis in a family facing this illness leaves many questions, among them being the duration and probable outcome of this illness.

The nurse, in caring for such patients and their families, should recognize at the outset of care that she must use all the resources available to her to gain as much knowledge as possible before her initial visit to the patient.

The following case history illustrates the complexity of the nursing problems and some of the nursing needs of the patient and his family.

BACKGROUND INFORMATION

A 37-year-old biophysicist was admitted to a local hospital for therapy of a metastatic neoplasm of unknown origin. The patient was well until November, 1963, when he had a bout of pleuritis, chest pain, and bronchitis which cleared uneventfully. In June, 1964, he noted hemoptysis. Chest x-ray showed a large mass adjacent to the right border of the lower mediastinum, possibly contiguous to the pericardium. Bronchoscopy and scalene node biopsy were performed and were negative. An angiogram suggested that the mass arose from

---

* Assistant Professor, University of Connecticut School of Nursing, Storrs.

the mediastinum. An exploratory thoracotomy at this time revealed that the tumor was actually arising from the pericardium. No biopsy of the lesion was obtained.

In August, 1964, when the patient was admitted to another local hospital, x-rays showed bilateral metastatic lesions in the lung fields. The patient received a course of nitrogen mustard therapy. Following this therapy, there was improvement and he was placed on maintenance chlorambucil therapy. The patient was aware of his illness and the plan of therapy.

Family history indicated that his mother had had a radical mastectomy ten years ago and his father had had a gastrectomy for cancer of the stomach fourteen years ago. Both parents were still living.

No allergic background was noted.

Physical examination revealed a pleasant white man in no apparent distress at rest, but experiencing severe pain in his left groin with slight motion. He was ashen gray in color, tall and thin.

FIRST ADMISSION TO X HOSPITAL

I met the patient for the first time the morning after his admission. He was lying on his left side and he told me that the pain in his left leg was again unbearable. Medication was given and I proceeded to make him comfortable. As I moved about, he told me he had worked in a hospital while going to school and it was there that he met his wife, who is a nurse. In giving him care, I learned that they have eight children ages 1 to 13 years. He was watching me very carefully and commenting on the routines for patient care elsewhere. Then, suddenly, he told me about his condition and the prognosis expected —"Six months, if I'm lucky." He said, "I never thought I would be praying for a lymphosarcoma but I am." I commented on his stoic acceptance of this diagnosis. It was then that I learned that the patient was a devout Catholic. He was here to receive therapy with the hope of a remission.

More x-rays were taken which showed a lesion in the left acetabulum, and biopsy revealed it to be a reticulum cell sarcoma. Of all lymphomas, this is perhaps the most malignant type. He was given Cytoxan 30 mg. per kg. intravenously.[3] A severe pancytopenia developed which was treated by transfusion of whole blood. Over the course of one week the patient's clinical status improved markedly. It was possible to decrease the dose of the prednisone he had been receiving and his need for narcotics became less. The patient became clinically very much better.

He was treated by physical therapy including range of motion and walking exercises for his left leg. Appropriate instructions were given for the use of crutches, and the patient was able, at the time of discharge, to walk on them for a distance of 100 feet before becoming dyspneic.

On the division where he was a patient, other personnel were aware of his diagnosis and what this meant in terms of his prognosis. The student nurse working with him during this admission found it difficult to establish a rapport because, as she put it, "He is a scientist and I am just a student." This student needed help in minimizing their differences in educational background and emphasizing patient relationships. The patient was being avoided by the young student nurse as well as by other nursing personnel because of his poor prognosis. This problem was at least partially solved by conferences with instructor, head nurse, physician, and psychiatrist who helped to bring feelings out in the open.

The patient would reminisce often about his family and expressed deep concern about their future and how they would fare without him. He spoke of the close family ties: how they attended church and social functions together, and when something happened to one member, all were concerned. Obviously they would be concerned now. He was worried also about the expense of a prolonged hospitalization.

The social service department and the availability of their service were explained to him, but for the present he felt he didn't need this service. His parish priest had discussed with him the community agencies that could and would help when, and if, needed. It was with the help of his parish priest that a housekeeper was found so that his wife could visit him. The visiting nurse service also had been explained.

On October 27, 1964, he was discharged. He was to be followed by his private physician and was instructed to continue taking the Cytoxan and to return daily to the hospital for radiation therapy. He appeared happy and said he "had a feeling of hope and something to go on."

INTERIM PRIOR TO SECOND ADMISSION

For a short time the patient remained asymptomatic. He enjoyed being with his family again and was working part time. His only complaint was that he tired very easily. He was evaluated for open heart surgery to remove the primary tumor, but a chest x-ray on December 8 revealed multiple, soft, round metastatic lesions that were too numerous to be removed by surgery.

On the day before Christmas the patient, for the first time, had a seizure, and Dilantin and phenobarbital therapy was begun. The medication controlled these attacks. At this time he was anointed by his parish priest.

Shortly after Christmas, he fell in his home and hit his head. A brain scan done at this time was normal. However, as a result of this fall the patient developed hemiparesis on his left side.

SECOND ADMISSION TO X HOSPITAL—JANUARY 18, 1965

On the morning of the 19th I was greeted by his wife who had spent an anxious night by his bedside. She left to make the hour's drive to see how their children had fared in her absence.

At this time the patient was responsive and oriented, but his senses seemed somewhat dulled. His chief complaints were difficulty in swallowing, hemiparesis of his left side, and shortness of breath. An intravenous infusion was started to replace the electrolytes he had lost through anorexia and vomiting. An electroencephalogram was done. Burr holes were made to rule out a subdural hematoma and in anticipation of x-ray therapy to the cerebrum.

A lumbar puncture produced xanthochromic fluid which contained 28 red blood cells. The opening pressure was 320 ml. of saline. The spinal fluid protein was elevated; this would substantiate a subdural hematoma. The procedure was well tolerated.

Nursing Care. The nursing care techniques involved were those used in caring for any obtunded person: suction at the bedside, airway attached to the head of the bed, turning, skin care, positioning, neurologic vital signs every hour. All the preventive and rehabilitative nursing techniques such as positioning, alignment, and exercises had to be done even in this gravely ill man. Where there is life, there is hope.

The patient experienced fear of choking. His anxiety was probably somewhat increased by the knowledge that any day might be his last. He seemed to be in a better state when someone was with him, and arrangements were made for a private duty nurse to be with him during the night.

I found that just by being myself I could be more effective in meeting his needs. It was necessary for me to make decisions for him when he was acutely ill, as to when to be turned, bathed, etc., but I carefully explained what I was doing and why. A nod or other signs told me he was at least aware of what I was doing. I, too, was deeply concerned about his prognosis and he knew I cared. (My feeling for him was doubtless made even deeper by my unconscious evaluation of him as high on the scale of social loss—see Glaser and Straus.[5])

On January 21 problems concerning urinary incontinence increased.

The patient was excreting large amounts of very light colored urine which he was unable to anticipate fully. Each of these incontinent incidents embarrassed him as it necessitated a complete change of bed linen. This problem was overcome quite easily by leaving a urinal in place and emptying it frequently. Whatever the cause, the incontinence improved and the next day he became brighter and less obtunded. This was the first note of encouragement in his second admission and we celebrated. The radio was playing and the atmosphere seemed more relaxed.

Four days passed before I saw him again. The change in his condition was remarkable; he appeared much improved, and the nursing care problems were different. One of the immediate problems was to coordinate his care with other departments so that he would be free to visit with his wife in the afternoons. His physical condition no longer demanded close attention. Since he had been so ill a few days before, now he could easily feel ignored. In the conferences with the nursing staff and others, a decision was made to visit him often.

He needed to be encouraged to use his left extremities which were regaining their lost function. Muscle setting exercises were prescribed. Most of what had to be done could be done by him alone, but he needed support and encouragement.

During this time I was able to know his wife better. Each afternoon she would come, always in a different outfit and looking nice. They had the afternoon free and I was asked to stay, if I had time! I knew that talking about plans would help their acceptance of them. It was also easier to talk to the patient when I knew what some of their thinking had been. I learned that his wife had made further inquiries and, for the present, their finances were in good order. The housekeeper was a "jewel," and with the help of good neighbors, all seemed well at home. They were not giving up hope. He would, in her presence, refer to "when I go back to work." He indicated to me later that he said this to make things easier for his wife. His wife was carrying on in a constructive, helpful way, and in doing so, she made a real contribution to the care that he received. Yet, on several occasions, she expressed feelings of guilt (as he had done on numerous occasions) because they did not come to X hospital sooner. "If we'd come here in the beginning, maybe...." It was important that she not take upon herself such a burden of guilt as this. I listened, but did not support her guilt. When she expressed these feelings, she was seeking reassurance that the right way was taken. By this time, both insisted that I call them by their first name and plan to come to see them.

As the patient improved, plans were again made for his discharge. He seemed anxious to return home, and because of his limited prognosis, it was decided that he would be discharged at the end of the week. Chemotherapy was to be continued while at home. Since he tired so easily, we talked about making arrangements for a bedroom on the first floor. Two days before he was supposed to go home, he had a spiking temperature. He reacted as if his whole world had shut in on him. Fortunately, on the day of discharge his temperature was normal and he was able to leave. The date was February 13, 1965.

FINAL ADMISSION

Three days after his previous discharge, the patient was readmitted to X Hospital. While he was home, he found that he tired more easily and was increasingly short of breath. It was impossible for him to sleep unless he was sitting up. His children were all ill with upper respiratory infections and he developed a productive cough and severe chest pain. He was seen in radiation therapy on February 16, 1965, and was transferred from there to the patient division.

An EKG performed on admission indicated that tachycardia had increased since his last reading on January 18, 1965. Shortness of breath was found to be due to increasing pleural effusion. Thoracentesis was done and a follow-up chest x-ray indicated that there was some reduction in the right pleural effusion, but there was still a large amout of effusion bilaterally. Also noted was extensive nodular disease throughout both lung fields.

On the morning following his admission, he was exhausted. I indicated surprise at seeing him back so soon and he said he had finally decided to "give up." What little hope he had three days ago was taken from him. He was too tired for his bath, but indicated a desire to have me stay with him. He was having more difficulty breathing and had assumed Fowler's position. I found that by arranging several pillows behind his back he was considerably more comfortable. He was quite apprehensive and told me he knew he would never be going home again.

On the following morning, he appeared less short of breath. He was still quite anxious and asked if I would accompany him to physical therapy. He was unable to take more than a few steps. That afternoon he started to run a low grade fever. There was no infectious organism present; the temperature was thought to be related to the tumor activity.

On February 18, 1965, a second thoracentesis was performed. A large amount of fluid was obtained from his right side; the effusion in his left side was worse. He told me that he thought the end was near. I tried to comfort him and spent a good deal of time just listening to him. The priest came in frequently to be with him, and the psychiatrist also visited.

From that day on, he and I never discussed his prognosis. We made a pact that while life was still in him we would discuss only things that were alive. We had many common interests: travel, literature, music, medicine, and children. We discussed his family at great lengths and he seemed very interested in what I would be doing in the future.

A closed thoracotomy was done on the 19th of February. The chest was drained and nitrogen mustard instilled, with excellent clinical results without accumulation of fluid on that side. However, fluid accumulated on the other side, and for this reason another chest tube was put in that area, fluid was withdrawn and nitrogen mustard instilled. However, the clinical response to this instillation of nitrogen mustard was not so marked as noted on the left side; fluid began to reaccumulate. The patient gradually went downhill.

His wife was spending as much time with her husband as she possibly could. She, too, realized that the end was near. They seemed to be reliving moments of the past and avoiding as much as possible any mention of the future. Their children visited and seemed to be a source of comfort to both of them.

On the day after the thoracotomy, there was a temperature elevation of 103°. Serosanguineous fluid was draining at the site of the tube insertion, and the fever was thought to be secondary to this. The leukocyte count was 1050. The patient began to experience severe chest pain, and the tube was pulled. His color was poor and it seemed to be an effort for him to speak. He was extremely apprehensive.

During the next two days, he developed oral moniliasis on the soft palate and right buccal mucosa. He was treated with nystatin and mouth wash. His leukocyte count was now 850. His physician was considering transfusion with white blood cells. He was cachexic and very anxious.

On February 24, 1965, he had massive diarrhea. The stool was positive for occult blood and Candida was noted in a specimen.

The last time I saw him was on February 26. I told him I would be back on Monday (this was Saturday) and he said he wouldn't be there. He asked me to continue praying for him, and told me he would always know that I would continue to care and hoped I would go to see his family.

An intercostal block of T5–9 was done on February 27 to relieve some of his pain. Within 10 minutes after the procedure he was feeling better. The next morning I learned he had a restless night and was failing rapidly. His blood pressure was unobtainable and his tachycardia was increasing. He died at 9 : 30.

CONCLUSIONS

1. Patients have basic needs, and the need for alleviating suffering both physical and mental is important in giving nursing care.
2. Religion can provide the motivation to live, to put one's house in order, to help his loved ones, and to die in peace.
3. A patient may be helped or hindered by the people around him, by their attitudes toward him, his family, and the illness, and their feelings about illness.
4. Patients become aware of our attitudes through our method of working with them.
5. Feelings about illness are an integral part of the meaning of illness to the ill patient; such feelings include fear, anxiety, loss of self-esteem, changing self-concept, loneliness, and dependency.
6. A patient is helped when the nurse takes the opportunity to learn how his family sees his illness and works with them for the good of the patient.
7. A nurse is helpful when she recognizes that she herself must be flexible enough to meet all sorts of problems, and that not only is there room for a variety of professional workers but that often the multiprofessional team is necessary.
8. The nurse should recognize also the need for a skillful evaluation of the personality structure of the patient as well as his condition at the outset of care and at suitable intervals thereafter.

REFERENCES

1. Best, Nelliana: Radiotherapy and the nurse. Am. J. Nursing, 50:140–143, 1950.
2. Brucker, E. A., and Glassy, F. J.: Primary reticulum cell sarcoma of the heart with review of the literature. Cancer, 8:921–931, 1955.
3. Calabresi, P., and Welch, A. D.: Chemotherapy of neoplastic disease. Ann. Rev. Med., 13:147–202, 1962.
4. Drummond, Eleanor E.: Impact of a father's illness. Am. J. Nursing, 64:89–91, 1964.
5. Glaser, B. G., and Strauss, A. L.: The social loss of dying patients. Am. J. Nursing, 64:119–121, 1964.
6. Musser, Ruth D., and Shubkagel, Betty Lou: Pharmacology and Therapeutics. 3rd Ed. New York, The Macmillan Co., 1965.
7. Saunders, Cicily: Should a Patient Know—? Nursing Times, pp. 994–995, Oct. 16, 1959.
8. Saunders, Cicily: Mental distress in the dying. Nursing Times, pp. 1067–1069, Oct. 30, 1959.
9. Towers, R. P., and Mulcahy, R.: Primary sarcoma of the pericardium. Brit. Heart J., 24:671–672, 1962.
10. Water, W. M.: Tumors of the heart and pericardium. Arch. Int. Med., 48:627-666, 1931.

470 Prospect St.
New Haven, Connecticut

Rationale of Nursing Care for Patients with Blood Dyscrasias

by BARBARA M. GURSKI, M.A.*

A blood dyscrasia is an alteration in the physiology of the blood. Dyscrasias may be of one of two types—congenital or acquired. The *congenital* alterations are generally due to the absence of the body's ability to produce one or more of the elements necessary for clotting, causing a bleeding tendency in the young child. Congenital dyscrasias generally allow the child to maintain the normal physiologic functions of cellular supply, but the ability is lacking to retain the blood when vascular injury occurs. Examples of congenital dyscrasias include hemophilia, the purpuras, and disorders affecting the prothrombin content.

Acquired dyscrasias are generally due to an acquired inability of the body to maintain a normal cycle of equilibrium between the production and the destruction of certain blood elements. The cellular structure most generally affected in the acquired dyscrasias is the erythrocyte. Reduction in the number of erythrocytes present in the circulation limits oxygen transportation to the cells. Without oxygen, the body cells have limited ability to utilize nutrients or carry on the metabolism that is necessary for their existence and activity. The acquired dyscrasias are generally active, progressive, symptomatic, and chronic. Among them are the various anemias, the leukemias, hemolytic jaundice, and the hemoglobinurias.

SYMPTOMS OF DYSCRASIAS IN RELATION TO NURSING CARE

The major symptoms are those that are due to a lessening of the body's ability to maintain the necessary cellular metabolism for energy, which in turn leads to a decrease in the body's potential for activity.

---

* Instructor, University of Connecticut School of Nursing, Storrs.

The symptoms which follow are a result of this lack as it affects specific systems in the body. The nursing care involved is centered about the physical care, prevention of complications, alleviation of symptoms, and teaching of the patient.

FATIGUE

The amount of activity an individual can undertake will be limited. The nurse must consider this in her ministrations to the patient. She should explain to the patient that the reason for the restriction in activity is to prevent overexertion, on the basis that the slower one works, the less the body's demand for nutrient needs, and so one can work longer. It should be emphasized that activity should be curtailed short of the point of fatigue, for once fatigue has set in it will take the body a longer period of time to regain its strength. The nurse can explain that frequent rest periods permit the body to recuperate to a point at which the nutrient supply satisfies the body demand, hence strength is regained.

The nurse can conserve the patient's strength by working slowly with him during any cooperative procedure, such as a bath. In addition, she should observe and ask the patient about his activity tolerance during any procedure and should arrange for his rest periods during the day according to his needs.

DYSPNEA

To prevent dyspnea, the nurse should be able to recognize the amount of activity the patient can tolerate before it begins. She should limit his daily activities to this level and assist him, as in bathing and shaving, when necessary. The patient can get relief from his symptoms by remaining in bed, because rest will result in a decreased oxygen demand by the body. He should be assisted into an orthopneic (upright) position so that he will have full lung expansion and, if ordered, oxygen should be administered so that he may inhale a higher oxygen concentration with less effort.

PALPITATION

An increase in the heart rate, and a consequent increase in the velocity of the blood flow, are common in the anemias, and they represent part of the body's effort to compensate for the lack of oxygen supply to the cells. Since the psyche is acutely aware of any change in the cardiac pace, the patient often becomes aware of the increased heart rate and suffers palpitations. Dyspnea is usually present at the same time, and for the same reason, and both conditions are treated by bed rest.

The sensation of palpitations can cause the patient to become distressed, and to ease the patient's apprehension, the nurse should explain why the heart is beating faster and how rest can reduce the palpitations or the velocity. If the apprehension continues, it is wise for the nurse to divert the patient's attention away from the sensation to other matters.

SENSITIVITY TO COLD

This is due to a constriction of the peripheral vascular bed which helps to maintain the needed nutrients and oxygen in the vital organs. The symptoms are similar to those of shock, but not so acute. With this peripheral vascular constriction, the patient is aware of any change in the atmospheric temperature. He is sensitive to the slightest breeze and is constantly trying to keep warm. The nurse should advise the patient to keep away from open windows and doors and to wear a sweater and socks, and should offer a blanket. She will generally refuse the patient's request for a hot water bottle or heating pad, explaining that these will dilate the peripheral vessels, taking away the blood from the vital centers and causing him to faint or feel dizzy.

FEVER

The fever that is sometimes seen in the patient with a dyscrasia may possibly be due to a failure in the nutrient supply to the hypothalamic area of the brain, where the body temperature is controlled, or to the general dehydration usually associated with dyscrasias.

The important nursing measures in caring for a febrile patient of this type are (1) to lower the elevated temperature in order to decrease the metabolic rate, and (2) to increase the fluid intake in order to supply the body heat with a conduction outlet to the atmosphere. The body temperature may be lowered by applying cooling sponges to the skin to induce heat loss. The sponges should be discontinued when the patient begins to shiver, because this additional muscular activity will produce more heat, thus defeating the purpose of the procedure. Antipyretic drugs such as aspirin may be administered if they are prescribed. These drugs act on the hypothalamic area to reduce the temperature and generally cause the patient to perspire during the temperature-lowering process. The body releases the fluid to transport the heat, and the nurse should be aware of this and try to keep the patient dry and avoid chilling. Fluid intake should be calculated in relation to fluid loss, and care must be taken not to overload the poorly functioning circulatory system.

BLEEDING TENDENCY

A bleeding tendency is the inability of the body to prevent whole blood loss, either in minute or large quantities.

The tendency is present in the purpuras and in the various abnormalities of blood coagulation which are due to deficiencies of particular blood factors, as in prothrombin deficiency and afibrinogenemia. In these conditions the bleeding is of two types: visible, which occurs subcutaneously or in the mucous membranes; or invisible, which occurs in the internal organs. Visible bleeding is usually minor, with minimal blood loss, unless a large vessel is involved. Generally, for visible bleeding, an application of ice to constrict the bleeding vessel or a prescribed topical application of some thrombin product to aid in coagulation at the site of an open wound may be initiated.

The nurse should urge the patient to be gentle about his mouth care, keeping the nose clean to limit the desire to manipulate it and blowing his nose gently so as not to rupture a fragile vessel in the nose. Care should be stressed in the use of sharp instruments such as cuticle scissors, straight razors, and knives. The nurse may stress other methods or instruments that could be substituted and that would yield the same results. She can caution the patient to use care when walking on slippery floors and loose mats so as to prevent falling. In caring for a child with a bleeding tendency, it is important to tell the mother to supervise the child's activities and curtail those that may traumatize.

The nurse may institute precautionary measures to reduce trauma in caring for the patient, such as keeping the patient's environment free of clutter, handling the patient's body gently, grasping the patient gently at the joints for any body manipulation, and limiting the number of injections the patient is receiving. She may prevent a hematoma from occurring at the injection site by applying pressure to the site for 3 to 5 minutes after an injection. If the patient is to receive multiple transfusions, the nurse may inquire of the doctor if the vein is to be kept open with some slow drip solution so that further punctures may be avoided. During the transfusion, the nurse should observe the patient for any adverse reactions which may indicate an incompatibility of blood types.

Invisible bleeding is suggested to the nurse by a change in the patient's vital signs and by traces of blood in the urine and stool. If hemorrhaging occurs, the patient is put to bed, the physician notified, and vital signs should be checked frequently. Profuse bleeding is treated by the administration of whole fresh blood which contains the factors necessary for coagulation. Narcotics are usually limited when there is bleeding because they may mask the pain associated with further bleeding.

The major responsibility of the nurse in caring for the patient with a bleeding tendency is to be alert to any change in his physical condition and to watch his skin, orifices, and excretions for bleeding so that when it occurs it can be reported and controlled early.

LOWERED BODY RESISTANCE

This is caused generally by a decrease in phagocytic leukocytes which the blood supplies, and in those chemical substances the blood conveys which are used for the body's defense against invading agents. This decline enhances the virulence of the bacteria in and on the patient. For this reason, the nurse teaches the patient to initiate meticulous hygienic measures. Both the patient and the nurse should be aware of the avenues of infection, such as hands, air, and clothing, so that precautions can be taken to prevent unnecessary exposure of the patient to pathogenic organisms which may be transmitted through these avenues. The nurse may assist the patient by adopting reverse precautions, that is, placing the patient in a private room, limiting visitors, and having all visitors and personnel entering the room wear gowns and masks. The principle here is to prevent the organisms from coming to the patient. If the nurse has some signs of bacterial invasion within herself, she should consider the patient's welfare and request reassignment until her condition abates. When an infection of some sort occurs in the patient, the nurse should note it and report it early in order that antibiotic therapy may be instituted.

GASTROINTESTINAL UPSETS

These are due to a decrease in the nutrition and oxygen supply to the gastrointestinal area, leading to sensitivity with resultant hyperactive responses such as anorexia, nausea, vomiting, and diarrhea. With anorexia, the patient should be encouraged to partake of food. The nurse can assist the patient by offering small, frequent feedings of easily masticated and easily digestible foods, consulting with him as to his likes and dislikes. Carbohydrates are limited because of their potential for decreasing the appetite and increasing flatulence. Foods with much roughage and drastic cathartics are avoided because they may injure already sensitive mucous membrane. The temperature of the food should not be too hot or too cold for the same reason.

When nausea and vomiting are present, food and fluid is restricted until the symptoms subside. If the vomiting persists, antiemetic drugs and intravenous therapy are started. The intravenous therapy is instituted to compensate for the loss of fluid and electrolytes through vomiting and to prevent dehydration. When the period of nausea and vomiting is over, the diet is slowly increased from liquid to soft foods to reduce the possibility of the reoccurrence of symptoms.

If diarrhea persists, it may be treated with prescribed antidiarrheal drugs, generally of opiate origin. The nurse should observe the stool for blood, undigested food, and tissue sloughings, and record the amount and type of stool that is passed. These observations are important in determining the condition of the bowel, and in the evaluation of the nutritive state of the patient and his electrolyte loss. Because of the irritating properties of the diarrheal stool, thorough anal cleansing after each evacuation is important to prevent excoriation.

NEUROLOGIC DYSFUNCTION

This results from the persistent and prolonged deficiency of nutrients and oxygen to the cellular structures in the nervous system. These dysfunctions may be categorized as minor and major.

Minor dysfunctions are tinnitus, spots before the eyes, vertigo, and drowsiness. These symptoms generally occur most vividly when the patient is in an erect position because this position favors the gravitational flow of blood from the brain, and the severity of the symptoms depends on the blood supply to the brain. For this reason the patient may favor the horizontal position in bed. Vertigo and drowsiness are the most distressing symptoms, and the patient should be cautioned about driving moving vehicles, smoking in bed, and taking care in walking downstairs. He should be taught to avoid sudden movements such as bending, getting out of bed, and turning, which may aggravate his symptoms by decreasing the blood supply to the brain suddenly. Bed rails should be up when there is loss of position sense, and items should be placed within the patient's reach to prevent exertion on his part.

Major neurologic dysfunctions are either spinal or cerebral. Symptoms of spinal cord involvement are disturbance in sphincter control and locomotor dysfunction. With the loss of sphincter control the bowel may exhibit incontinence or obstipation, and the bladder incontinence and retention. Bowel care will consist of prevention of obstipation through some dietary means, or the use of very mild laxatives or enemas. Bladder retention or incontinence is treated by the insertion of a retaining catheter. With incontinence of either bowel or bladder or possibly both, the nurse should initiate good skin care to prevent tissue breakdown.

Motor and sensory dysfunction require that the nurse take precautions in applying heat. With an increase in motor loss there is a decrease in patient initiated movements so that passive exercises should be religiously adhered to, in order to maintain muscle tone. Frequent change of the patient's position and good skin care at pressure sites are important in preventing decubitus formation, for these individuals have poor peripheral circulation with undernourished tissue, which enhances breakdown. Once a decubitus is formed in these patients it is difficult to heal.

Cerebral symptoms include loss of memory, diminution of intellectual capacity, depression, and clumsiness of fine movements. These symptoms are similar to those exhibited by patients with chronic brain degeneration or senility. In this situation, the nurse should be prepared to explain the procedures and the reasons for them repeatedly each time they are done. The nurse should be willing to carry on a conversation with the patient, allowing him to set the pace and the topic. The patient may have a flight of ideas but the nurse should not force him to concentrate on one topic, because this may be impossible.

Any tasks the nurse requires of the patient should be simple, with simple instructions requiring a minimum of time. The amount of supervision the patient needs will depend on his mental status. Any task requiring fine movements, such as sewing, or concentration, such as playing cards, is avoided and replaced by tasks or activities the patient can handle. This patient needs a calm and patient nurse and a calm environment for he is easily frustrated.

CONCLUSIONS

The patient with an active and progressive blood dyscrasia has limited physical and mental abilities due basically to a decrease in the ability of the blood to perform its function of carrying nutrients and oxygen to the cells. The severity of the symptoms and the degree to which they may progress depend on the cause of the disease and at what stage of the disease therapy was instituted.

The symptoms mentioned above generally are present in all active and progressive dyscrasias. Any dyscrasia with a decrease in erythrocytes evidences the symptoms caused by a decrease in the oxygen supply to the body, as is found in leukemia, pernicious anemia, and sickle cell anemia. In Hodgkin's disease, the symptoms are caused by pressure from enlarged nodes. In polycythemia vera, they result from engorged vessels. In essence, the nursing care of patients with all blood dyscrasias is basically similar.

These conditions are generally chronic and require lifelong therapy with periods of hospitalization. Both economic and psychologic adjustments must be made by the patient and the family. They may need assistance in setting definite physical, social, and economic goals. The patient has to be taught proper dietary needs for his condition and how to use his medications.

The four broad objectives of nursing care for the patients with progressive blood dyscrasias are: (1) to meet the patient's physical requirements by decreasing metabolic needs and preventing complications; (2) to carry out nursing responsibilities associated with medical therapy; (3) to establish a relationship with the patient through which he may feel supported; (4) to be alert to any change in the patient's condition which may indicate a need for a change in therapy or in nursing care.

REFERENCES

1. The Anemias. Eli Lilly and Company, Indianapolis, Indiana.
2. Brodish, Mary Stone: The nurse's role in the care of children with acute leukemia. Am. J. Nursing, 58:1572–1574, 1958.
3. Wintrobe, M. M.: Blood dyscrasias. Am. J. Nursing, 60:496–500, 1960.

461 Burritt St.
New Britain, Connecticut

The Role of the School Nurse in the Support of Children with Certain Cardiovascular Disorders

by HELEN T. WATSON, M.S.*

THE ROLE OF THE PROFESSIONAL NURSE IN THE SCHOOL SETTING

According to the National League for Nursing,[4] the professional nurse's ability to serve most adequately within the school setting, in contacts with students, school staff, and parents, is dependent upon basic preparation for professional nursing and additional preparation that enables her to:

1. Utilize concepts of human growth, development, and behavior in the milieu of the school health program.

2. Recognize developmental and health needs of pupils and students, especially in relation to prevention, detection, and treatment, which must influence educational programing.

3. Utilize existing services for children and youth and spearhead the development of additional services when indicated by the needs of the school health program.

4. Comprehend the nature of the educational setting in which the school nurse must work in collaboration with others from different professional disciplines.

5. Select and use processes appropriate to the role assumed by the school nurse.

It is important that the nurse working in an educational setting understand her role and be able to communicate it effectively to students, school staff members, parents, and others in the community. The present

---

* Assistant Professor, School of Nursing, University of Connecticut, Storrs.

paper offers an approach to a special problem in nursing in the school setting, namely, the process of evaluating, diagnosing, and intervening in incipient rheumatic heart disease and also of fostering the attainment and maintenance of equilibrium among students with cardiac defects.

To provide for effective intervention in cases of students with rheumatic fever or those who have medical histories indicating predispositions toward rheumatic fever, the nurse practitioner must be competent in her ability to assess, as described by McCain[6]; to reconnoiter, as discussed by Dr. Katherine Nelson during the Regional Workshops of 1961, sponsored by ANA, or to evaluate, diagnose, and intervene according to Rogers.[8] The three authors mentioned have been among the practitioners who have provided, through recent publications, bases for a definition of nursing which covers the primary function of professional nurses working in industrial and educational settings.

In speaking of fostering the attainment and maintenance of equilibrium as related to cardiac defects, the term "equilibrium" is used here to identify an optimum state of adjustment by the individual to the internal and external forces created by certain heart defects. This concept of the nurse's role in the educational setting is supported by Rogers in her statement on professional nursing as the process by which a body of scientific knowledge or nursing science "is used for the purpose of assisting human beings to achieve maximum health, within each person's potential, consistent with the scope and objectives of learned professional nursing."[8]

In the educational setting at the elementary school level the nurse has a responsibility for implementing this process primarily in relation to pupils and teachers together with school administrators and parents. At the secondary school level she is more directly involved with students and other pupil personnel workers, while at the college level her contacts are almost entirely with the students.

In any event the process involves two major assessments. The first is assessing the status of the student in terms of minimum to maximum well-being. To do this the nurse utilizes, in collaboration with others, her knowledge and competence in nursing for guidance toward the achievement of the full health and educational potential of each student. The second assessment is to decide upon and implement alternatives based on principles of prediction. These two assessments are part of the on-going process of utilizing scientific knowledge for the purpose of assisting human beings to achieve an equilibrium in the terms described above. This process must be dynamic in that the practitioner must constantly modify and change the major assessments encompassed.

THE NURSE'S ROLE IN REGISTRATION AND HISTORY-TAKING

When registering a child for admission to school, parents or guardians are expected to comply with admission requirements as regulated by state statutes or local decisions. In most instances birth certificates, evidence of certain inoculations, and health histories are required. The importance of accurate health history-taking cannot be overestimated, since schools have a legal responsibility for the welfare of pupils during the time of their attendance at school. The nurse is usually responsible for obtaining the health histories for the cumulative health records which the school keeps for each student. With cardiovascular conditions in mind, the school nurse conducts the registration interview in such a manner that facts concerning the frequency of throat or upper respiratory infections are brought out, as well as any previous medical evaluations having implications for cardiovascular disorders.

Even when medical attention has been infrequent or nonexistent since immediately after birth, the nurse uses her observational abilities to note any symptoms that may be indicative of infections that may precede rheumatic fever, of rheumatic fever itself, or of heart defects. This means that she looks for any signs of cyanosis of the epidermis in general, and the lips and fingernail beds in particular. She evaluates any rhythmic or regular behavior patterns which might be considered tics. A general assessment of physical stamina is also made.

Any histories or symptoms that suggest the possibility of these cardiovascular disorders should be identified so that follow-up functions can be activated immediately. This means helping parents plan for needed medical evaluations as soon as possible.

WHAT THE SCHOOL NURSE NEEDS TO KNOW IN ORDER TO ASSESS AND DEAL WITH CARDIOVASCULAR DISORDERS

In order to evaluate, diagnose, and intervene effectively in cases of cardiovascular disorders among school children, the school nurse must know the essential scientific facts about the extent and the effects of these disorders. In particular she must be aware of their prevalence among children, their causes and possible prevention, the extent of the disability caused by them, the results of research and experience in their management, and the internal and external manifestations of disequilibrium precipitated by them.

PREVALENCE OF CERTAIN CARDIOVASCULAR DISORDERS AMONG CHILDREN AND YOUTH

According to the American Heart Association,[1a] there is at least one child with heart disease in almost every classroom in the schools of this country each year. The Association has estimated[1c] that 30,000 to 40,000 infants are born in the United States with congenital heart defects each year. This number can be reasonably expected to increase as physicians utilize newer techniques for detecting such defects.

About one million Americans have rheumatic fever. It, together with rheumatic heart disease, is responsible for more handicapping illness in children and youth than is any other disease. These two disorders make up about two-thirds of all heart diseases in children, especially in the age range of 5 to 15.

ETIOLOGY AND COURSE OF RHEUMATIC FEVER AND RHEUMATIC HEART DISEASE

Although the immediate cause of rheumatic fever is unknown, it usually is preceded by nose and throat infections caused by organisms of the streptococcus family. As many as three streptococcal infections out of one hundred are followed by rheumatic fever. For the individual who has had one attack of rheumatic fever, the chances of recurrence are greatly increased. Examples of the types of infections that precede rheumatic fever are "strep" sore throat, tonsillitis, some ear infections, and scarlet fever.

The onset of rheumatic fever frequently begins about two to four weeks after the streptococcal infection has disappeared. While it should be stressed that every "strep" sore throat or infection is not followed by rheumatic fever, it should also be noted that some children can have "strep" infections without sore throats. Although rheumatic fever is not considered contagious, the streptococcal infection that precedes it is contagious.

Rheumatic fever may affect any part of the body, and often affects the heart, joints, blood vessels, skin, or brain. Each recurring attack of rheumatic fever increases the risk of damage to the heart. This damage may have serious or even fatal results, although the effects on other parts of the body are temporary in most cases. Attacks of rheumatic fever can last for weeks, months, or sometimes years. Its disappearance is not always permanent.

Rheumatic fever tends to run in families, but it has not been established whether this is due to hereditary or environmental factors. Rheumatic heart disease which is caused by rheumatic fever is the result of inflammation and scarring of the heart muscle and heart valves. This scarring may interfere with the vital work of the heart in pumping the body's blood supply.

Implications for the Nurse. The preceding facts have many implications for school nursing practice. For example, the school nurse will need to give leadership and direction to the formulation of school health policies designed to prevent the spread of possible streptococcal infections and facilitate their identification. Such policies might encourage those with sore throats to stay at home and seek medical advice, permit participation in a plan for throat cultures or penicillin prophylaxis in appropriate cases which have been predetermined by medical advice, and provide for adequate follow-up measures by the school nurse in instances of repeated attacks of sore throats or upper respiratory infections.

If school health policies include provisions for the taking of throat cultures, care in taking them cannot be overemphasized. A good technique for the school nurse is to see that the side of the swab comes down across the tonsil or tonsillar fossa on one side, the tip touching the posterior pharyngeal wall as it comes across the throat, and the other side of the swab touching the other tonsil or tonsillar fossa as it comes up, completing the "down-across-up" movement.[7]

THE NATURE OF CONGENITAL HEART DEFECTS

The cause of congenital heart defects or congenital heart disease is generally unknown. Regardless of which term is used, these kinds of abnormalities in infants are recognized as structural defects which occur at some point in the development of the heart or major vessels before birth. There are many types of congenital heart defects, which may occur alone or in combination with others. The most common defects with which infants survive are the abnormal openings and obstructions which may impair the child's circulatory system and hamper his growth and energy, for example, patent ductus arteriosus, atrial septal defect, and the combination of defects known as the tetralogy of Fallot.

THE EXTENT OF DISABILITY CAUSED BY THESE CARDIOVASCULAR CONDITIONS AMONG SCHOOL AGE CHILDREN AND YOUTH

According to the American Heart Association,[1a] about one-third of children with rheumatic fever recover completely without obvious heart damage. Another third may have some symptoms of cardiac damage but are not prevented from leading normal or almost normal lives. The remaining third of these children, who in most instances have had more than one rheumatic infection, develop heart disease serious enough to require special long-term planning. Generally the children in this latter group need home instruction for a considerable period of time.

Of the 30,000 to 40,000 children estimated as being born annually with congenital heart defects, about 75 to 80% can be helped by surgery.[1c] The objective of surgery is to restore circulation by repairing or partially repairing the defective part of the heart or blood vessel. The nurse should follow closely the progress of children who had had heart surgery, and should discuss with the parents, and with their approval with the physician, provisions for continuation of school work during convalescence.

When the school nurse becomes aware of the existence of cardiac defects in any students, parental permission to communicate with the private physician concerning adjustments to be made in the school program for such pupils should be sought immediately. While many of these children and youth may be required to observe only minor limitations regarding the extent of their physical activities, others may be limited to the minimum amount of physical exertion necessary to attend school classes.

RESULTS OF RESEARCH AND EXPERIENCE IN THE MANAGEMENT OF CARDIOVASCULAR DISORDERS IN CHILDREN AND YOUTH

Research and experience governing the everyday management of children and youth with cardiovascular disorders of the type under discussion continue to increase the possibility of these children and youth living normal or near normal lives.

The greatest progress in reducing the incidence of serious heart damage among children and youth has resulted from the concerted efforts of conscientious workers in the fields of medical and other research. Their efforts have provided the basis for the concept of rheumatic fever prophylaxis which has received widespread acceptance among medical practitioners during the past two decades. One such outstanding program is Connecticut's Rheumatic Fever Prevention Program which makes penicillin available for the prevention of recurrences of rheumatic fever at low cost to rheumatic fever patients through their physicians. The plan was developed with the leadership of the Connecticut Heart Association and cooperation of the Connecticut Pharmaceutical Association in June of 1955 and received the endorsement of the Connecticut State Medical Society and the Connecticut State Department of Health as the plan became more clearly defined. The program incorporates policies to provide careful controls over the distribution of low cost prophylactic medication and accurate statistical information for a study of the status of rheumatic fever in Connecticut.[9]

Following a successful demonstration of the value of rapid reporting of positive (Group A streptococcus) throat cultures in the control of streptococcal infections, the Connecticut State Department of Health and

CHILDREN WITH CARDIOVASCULAR DISORDERS 37

the Connecticut Heart Association endorsed a joint statement of recommendations for the treatment of cases and management of contacts affected by Group A streptococal infections.[7] The statement was prepared and issued by the Connecticut Heart Association in 1965 to all physicians and schools nurses in the state.

The school nurse must be familiar enough with the surgical and medical treatment of congenital heart defects to know the difference it makes to the child or youth so affected. By surgery, the malformed part of the heart or blood vessel may be repaired so as to correct the defect completely or partially, causing the circulation to become normal or near normal. Medical treatment is sometimes an alternative to surgery but cannot repair the original defect causing the symptoms. In the latter instances, the nurse must regularly ascertain that the pupil and his parents are aware of the need for continuous contact with their physician.

THE NURSE'S ROLE IN INSTANCES OF DISEQUILIBRIUM ON THE PART OF CHILDREN WITH CARDIOVASCULAR DISEASES

Internal and external manifestations of disequilibrium, or lack of adjustment, on the part of children and youth with established diagnoses of cardiovascular disease represent a critical challenge to the school nurse. Such circumstances demand professional competence in the utilization of nursing science to assist these students toward maximum achievement in keeping with their potential. The nursing practitioner must have knowledge and understanding of the attainment of equilibrium in order to be able to discern and assess a state of disequilibrium. Any plan of appropriate intervention must be based on such discernment.

Specifically, the school nurse must be able to help children and youth to accept their cardiovascular limitations in a positive manner. The extent to which they can engage in the activities of their peers should be stressed. The nurse can provide physicians with lists of activities described by physical education teachers so that they can indicate which activities their patients can engage in without jeopardizing their cardiovascular conditions.

The nurse should stress the need for these children to be included in the regular school classes and programs whenever possible. This can be accomplished through her sharing in the in-service education planning for all school staff members and in case conferences with other pupil personnel workers such as guidance counselors.

In her health counseling with parents of children whose cardiovascular conditions are being followed up, the nurse must be sensitive to their anxieties and fears for the everyday health hazards confronted by their children. She therefore supports the recommendation of physicians for full therapeutic dosages of penicillin or other antibiotics in the event of operative procedures such as tooth extractions or any dental treatment which breaks the gums, removal of tonsils and adenoids or any other procedure in the mouth, nose, or throat area, and surgery of the gastrointestinal, genital, or urinary tracts. Her support in these respects should be realistic, and her concern for being as positive as possible should not overshadow the necessity of observing medical precautions when common childhood diseases are being faced.

When the school nurse discerns what she assesses as signs of internal disequilibrium such as anxiety, projection, and overprotection in teachers who have children with cardiovascular conditions in their classrooms, she uses educational approaches to changing these attitudes and behavior.

Educational and vocational guidance for these children begins in an earlier grade than for other children. Their intellectual potential should be stimulated to the full since jobs that conserve strength tend to require more educational preparation.

The success of the nurse's efforts to establish equilibrium where disequilibrium exists can be discerned by behavior indicative of acceptance of children with these conditions by themselves, their parents, their teachers, and their peers.

REFERENCES

1. American Heart Association, 44 East 23rd St., New York City: (a) What the Classroom Teacher Should Know and Do About Children with Heart Disease (1958); (b) Home Care of the Child with Rheumatic Fever (1963); (c) If Your Child Has a Congenital Heart Defect (1960); (d) Diagnosis of Congenital Cardiac Defects in General Practice (1961); (e) Now You Can Protect Your Child Against Rheumatic Fever.
2. Blakeslee, A. L.: How to Live with Heart Trouble. Public Affairs Pamphlet No. 184, Public Affairs Committee, Inc., New York.
3. Smiley, Lyda: Health records for school children. Am. J. Nursing, 60:18-20, 1960.
4. Florentine, Helen G.: The Preparation and the Role of the Nurses in School Health Programs. National League for Nursing, 1962.
5. Johnson, Dorothy E.: The significance of nursing care. Am. J. Nursing, 61:63-66, Nov., 1961.
6. McCain, R. Faye: Nursing by assessment—not intuition. Am. J. Nursing, 65:82-84, April, 1965.
7. The Rheumatic Fever Committee Recommendations for (I) Treatment of Cases of Group A Streptococcal Infection. (II) Management of contacts—a joint statement of The Connecticut Heart Association and the Connecticut State Department of Health. Connecticut Heart Association, 65 Wethersfield Avenue, Hartford, Conn.
8. Rogers, Martha E.: Some comments on the theoretical basis of nursing practice. Nursing Sc., 1:11-13, 60-61, 1963.
9. Spinelli, N. P. R., Brown, H. A., and Lavnikevick, N. J.: Operation of a cooperative state-wide rheumatic fever prevention program. Am. J. Pub. Health, 51:256-260, 1961.

Impaired Pulmonary Circulation Due to Pulmonary Emphysema

by HELEN CHUAN, M.N.*

A middle-aged man was sitting in a wheel chair waiting to be admitted to the hospital. He looked chronically ill, his respirations were labored and wheezy, and he appeared to have kyphosis. These symptoms are not uncommon today, and are often evidence of the presence of pulmonary emphysema.

The incidence of pulmonary emphysema has been increasing in recent years. The following facts may be responsible for its actual increase or its more frequent recognition: the increasing age of the population, the greater awareness of the public, and the physician's ability to diagnose with the aid of advanced laboratory techniques. The disease is rated as second on the National Health Disability list. Its impact on the economy and on social welfare is serious; therefore, nurses must be prepared to give effective nursing care, and to do this, the pathophysiologic changes occurring must be comprehended.

There are many predisposing factors. Cigarette smoking is believed by many authorities to be the leading cause of the development of chronic bronchitis and pulmonary emphysema. Other contributing factors are air pollution, chronic upper respiratory infections, asthma, congenital anomalies of the thoracic and pulmonary structures, hypersensitivity of the lung tissue, and occupational hazards.

PATHOLOGIC AND PHYSIOLOGIC CHANGES IN CHRONIC BRONCHITIS AND PULMONARY EMPHYSEMA

Chronic irritation causes hypertrophy of the smooth muscles of the bronchial wall, hyperplasia of the goblet cells, and loss of cilia and their function, resulting in narrowing, thickening, and fibrosis of the

---

* Instructor in Nursing, University of Connecticut School of Nursing, Storrs.

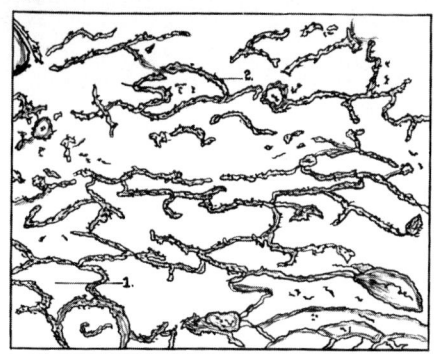

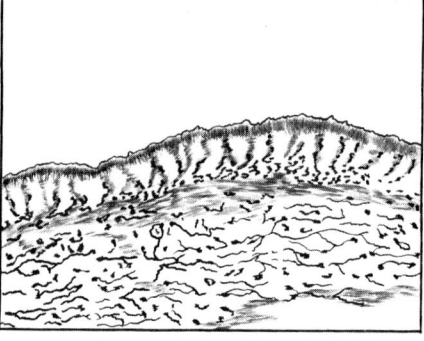

Figure 1. Diagrammatic illustration of normal lung structure. 1, Alveolus. 2, Alveolar septum.
Figure 2. Diagrammatic illustration of normal bronchial epithelium:

bronchial passages and producing the symptoms of dyspnea, wheezing, cough, and hypersecretion. Emphysema will inevitably develop after a period of chronic bronchitis. Air obstruction and air resistance produce distention of the alveoli, rupture and loss of alveolar septa, thickening of the alveolar walls, and reduction of the vascular channels; these in turn result in ventilatory deficiency which leads to CO_2 retention and arterial oxygen unsaturation. Pulmonary hypertension, pulmonary acidosis, polycythemia, and cor pulmonale may follow.

Figures 1 through 4 show in diagrammatic fashion the changes that take place in the alveoli and the resultant appearance of the bronchial epithelium. Compare Figures 1 and 2 with 3 and 4. Notice the enlarged alveoli, absence of the alveolar septa, and thickening of the alveolar walls in emphysema.

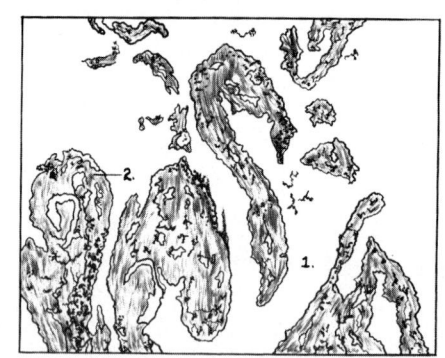

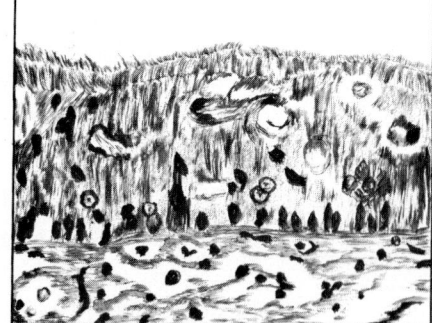

Figure 3. Diagrammatic illustration of the structure of an emphysematous lung. 1, Alveolus. 2, Alveolar septum.
Figure 4. Diagrammatic illustration showing hyperplasia of the bronchial epithelium.
(Illustrations modified from photographs by Dr. Oscar Auerbach.)

DIAGNOSTIC AND LABORATORY TESTS

In addition to recognizing the pathologic and physiologic changes, nurses should be familiar with the various diagnostic and laboratory tests and be able to correlate the findings with the patient's clinical condition. The results of the laboratory findings not only indicate the patient's condition, but also help to predict his response to treatment.

1. **Chest X-Ray.** This demonstrates increased anterior-posterior diameter of the chest, flattened and depressed diaphragm, increased radiolucency of the lungs, and, in severe cases, enlargement of the heart.

2. **Pulmonary Function Tests.** These enable the physician to assess the degree of emphysema more accurately than do radiographic and physical examinations.

   a. *Vital Capacity.* This represents the volume of air expired in the fullest possible expiration after the deepest possible inspiration. This volume is usually less than normal in emphysema owing to the flattened diaphragm and the loss of recoil action of the lung tissue.

   b. *Timed Vital Capacity.* A much longer time of expiration is demonstrated in the emphysematous patient. This is due to airway obstruction, bronchospasm, loss of tissue elasticity, bronchial collapse, restriction of the chest, and other factors.

   c. *Residual Volume or Residual Air.* This is the air volume remaining in the lungs after the fullest possible expiration. This volume is found greatly increased in the emphysematous patient because of the enlarged air sacs, fibrosis of the lung tissue, impaired gas diffusion, and airway obstruction.

3. **Arterial Blood Gases Tests.** These studies are essential in the evaluation of the patient's condition and in the determination of therapy.

LABORATORY FINDINGS IN EMPHYSEMA

Test	Normal	Patient
Total lung capacity	3.5–6.5 Liters	5.3 Liters
Vital capacity	2.5–5.0 "	1.5 "
Residual volume	0.8–1.5 "	3.23 "
Total vital capacity time		9.4 sec.
Physiologic dead space	0.150 Liters	1.76 Liters
Arterial oxygen pressure	95 mm. Hg	43 mm. Hg
Arterial oxygen saturation	94%	87%
Arterial CO_2 pressure	35–45 mm. Hg	73 mm. Hg
Arterial blood pH	7.35–7.45	7.15
Hematocrit	45–50%	61%
Bicarbonate	25.1–30.5 mEq/L.	32.7 mEq./L.

The arterial blood gas studies include oxygen saturation, carbon dioxide content, carbon dioxide tension, arterial blood pH and bicarbonate level. As a result of ventilatory deficiency, the oxygen saturation decreases, carbon dioxide content increases and carbon dioxide tension becomes elevated. The effect of the gaseous disturbances on the patient will be discussed later.

The table on page 41 shows normal laboratory findings as compared with those for an actual emphysematous patient.

COMPLICATIONS AND TREATMENT

Only the common complications will be discussed.

RESPIRATORY INFECTION

Nurses must be on the alert at all times for signs of increased dyspnea, cough, secretion, and elevated temperature. Emphysematous patients are extremely susceptible to respiratory infections. The common organisms found in cultures of sputum are pneumococci, *H. influenzae, Staphylococcus aureus,* and Group A hemolytic streptococcus. Respiratory infection can lead to serious complications if medical treatment is delayed.

Hypersensitivity to respiratory infection in emphysema is probably due to the many changes in the cardiopulmonary system already mentioned, such as the loss of cilia and their function, inflammation of the bronchial walls, hypersecretion, increased dead air space, etc.

Respiratory infection undoubtedly will increase ventilatory deficiency and cause further gas exchange impairment by means of further obliteration of the bronchioles and alveoli. Ulceration, destruction, and scarring of the alveolar septa which could lead to pulmonary acidosis and death may ensue. Therefore, any sign of a respiratory infection calls for immediate medical attention. Antibiotic therapy, oxygen therapy, and inhalation therapy are the usual treatments of choice.

RESPIRATORY ACIDOSIS OR CARBON DIOXIDE NARCOSIS

The study of oxygen saturation, carbon dioxide content, carbon dioxide tension, and pH of the arterial blood plus the bicarbonate level is necessary in the determination of pulmonary acidosis. The patient is said to be in pulmonary acidosis when his CO_2 is above 42 mm. Hg, his arterial blood pH is below 7.35, and his oxygen saturation is below 85%.

Besides the expected signs and symptoms one finds in an acute emphysematous patient, the nurse may also observe mental disturbance and psychotic behavior before the patient goes into semicoma and coma. Cerebral anoxia and cerebral ischemia may play an important part in this.

Impairment of gas exchange is often exaggerated by respiratory infection, as stated before; however, other factors should not be ignored, such as increased air stagnation, diminished pulmonary capillary bed, scarring of pulmonary tissue, and decreased permeability due to this scarring.

The respiratory embarrassment must be corrected before respiratory arrest occurs. The treatment, of course, is aimed at ventilatory improvement. This is best accomplished by a skilled health team (physician, nurses, oxygen therapist, laboratory technician) and the cooperation of the patient.

The treatment usually consists of:

a. *Antibiotic therapy* to combat infection.

b. *Antibronchospasm* therapy via aerosol.

c. *Cortisone therapy* may also be used to reduce bronchospasm and bronchial inflammation.

d. *Reduction of bronchial secretions* by means of aerosol detergents to reduce surface tension, thus thinning the secretions to facilitate easier expectoration. Postural drainage is another method of eliminating secretions if it can be tolerated by the patient. Endotracheal suction is used routinely in unconscious patients and patients too ill to expectorate.

e. *Exercise and physical therapy* to encourage the patient to expire as fully as possible, to reduce residual volume and improve pulmonary ventilation by using the abdominal muscles. This can be done by placing a sandbag or a book on the patient's abdomen and watching the rise and fall of the abdomen during breathing. However, this exercise is not advisable for all patients. Those who are extremely hypoxic and unable to undertake any activity without being exhausted should not be encouraged to perform this exercise.

f. *Oxygen therapy.* The administration of oxygen to an emphysematous patient requires the supervision of a pulmonary specialist. Since the respiratory center becomes insensitive to the abnormally high CO_2 content in the arterial blood, the carotid body begins to compensate in order to restore the regular respiratory rate. The carotid body is only stimulated when hypoxia is present. Administration of concentrated oxygen could lead to arrest of carotid body function and thus create a more serious situation in which the patient becomes sluggish, lethargic, and unconscious. Death may follow.

Careful administration of oxygen with aerosol detergent under intermittent positive pressure (see p.144) is very valuable in treating pulmonary acidotic patients. It improves ventilation, reduces airway obstruction, and stimulates expectoration.

g. *Tracheostomy* may be a necessary procedure for patients in acute respiratory distress. It allows more adequate aspiration of bronchial secretions, and ventilation can be improved by attaching the IPPB machine to the tracheostomy site.

COR PULMONALE

Essentially, this is a cardiac failure produced by lung disease and pulmonary hypertension, rather than by cardiac disease per se. Most authorities agree that pulmonary hypertension is caused by arterial hypoxia and that cor pulmonale is a result of pulmonary hypertension (see diagram).

The cardiac impairment occurs in the right heart. The signs and symptoms include right ventricular enlargement, distended neck veins, increased venous pressure, increased circulation time, central cyanosis, peripheral edema, enlarged liver, ascites, and hydrothorax, all of which may or may not appear, depending on the degree of severity.

Sequence of Physiologic Changes in Chronic Pulmonary Emphysema

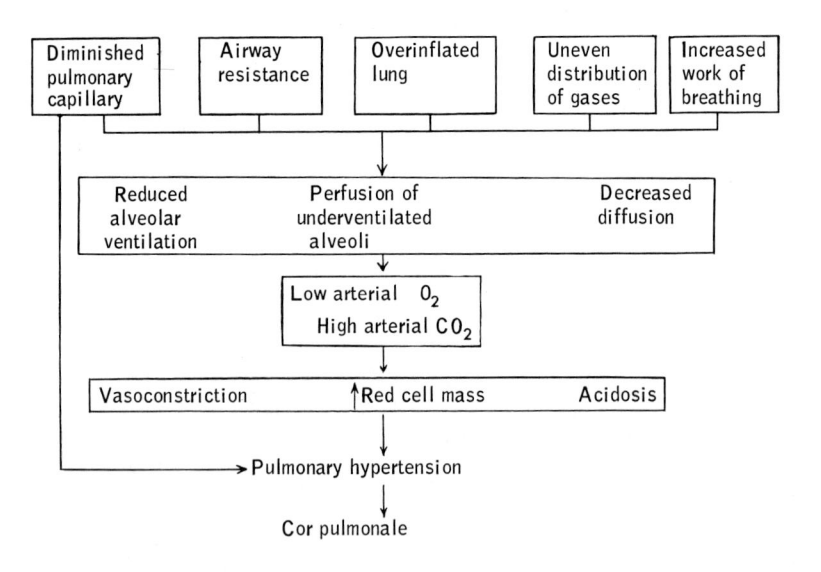

```
┌─────────────┬───────────┬─────────────┬─────────────┬─────────────┐
│ Diminished  │ Airway    │ Overinflated│ Uneven      │ Increased   │
│ pulmonary   │ resistance│ lung        │ distribution│ work of     │
│ capillary   │           │             │ of gases    │ breathing   │
└─────────────┴───────────┴─────────────┴─────────────┴─────────────┘
                                │
                                ▼
        ┌──────────────────────────────────────────────────┐
        │  Reduced       Perfusion of        Decreased     │
        │  alveolar      underventilated     diffusion     │
        │  ventilation   alveoli                           │
        └──────────────────────────────────────────────────┘
                                │
                                ▼
                    ┌──────────────────────┐
                    │ Low arterial  O₂     │
                    │ High arterial CO₂    │
                    └──────────────────────┘
                                │
                                ▼
        ┌──────────────────┬──────────────────┬──────────────┐
        │ Vasoconstriction │ ↑Red cell mass   │ Acidosis     │
        └──────────────────┴──────────────────┴──────────────┘
                                │
                                ▼
                  → Pulmonary hypertension
                                │
                                ▼
                          Cor pulmonale
```

Diagram from *Chronic Obstructive Pulmonary Emphysema*, published by the National Tuberculosis Association, p. 16.

In cor pulmonale the cardiac impairment is reversible. When pulmonary hypertension is relieved, symptoms of cardiac failure also diminish. Therefore, the chief concern in treating cor pulmonale is aimed toward the relief of pulmonary hypertension, which is reduced when ventilation is improved. Thus all the methods of improving ventilation that have been mentioned before would apply here. The usual treatments for heart failure may also be used in these cases, such as digitalization, diet therapy, and diuretic therapy.

POLYCYTHEMIA

Polycythemia is expected among patients with cor pulmonale. When chronic arterial hypoxia exists, the marrow is stimulated to produce more red blood cells to compensate. However, the presence of polycythemia creates higher venous pressure and pulmonary hypertension; therefore, phlebotomy is done routinely when the hematocrit reaches 55 per cent or more.

Other complications arising from pulmonary emphysema may include pneumothorax, peptic ulcer, pulmonary thrombosis and embolus, and arteriosclerotic hypertensive heart disease. These will not be discussed here.

CONCLUSIONS

Pulmonary emphysema is a progressive, destructive, and irreversible disease. Medical treatment and nursing care are aimed toward prevention of complications and further deterioration. The nurse's role in the prevention of respiratory infection and maintenance of adequate ventilation is essential.

Rehabilitation depends upon the patient's condition. Early detection and well planned treatment help many patients back to their former employment and years of fairly comfortable life.

ACKNOWLEDGMENT

Art work for this paper was done by Elaine C. Raymond, M.A.

REFERENCES

Beeson, P. B., and McDermott, W.: Cecil-Loeb Textbook of Medicine, 11th Ed. Philadelphia, W. B. Saunders Co., 1963.

Hass, Albert: The Application of Physical Medicine and Rehabilitation to Emphysema Patients. The Institute of Physical Medicine and Rehabilitation, New York University Medical Center, 1963.

Hass, Albert: Essentials of Living with Pulmonary Emphysema. The Institute of Physical Medicine and Rehabilitation, New York University Medical Center, 1963.
MacBryde, C. M.: Signs and Symptoms. 4th Ed. Philadelphia, J. B. Lippincott Co., 1964.
Orie, N. G. M.: Bronchitis. Netherland Royal Vangorcum, 1961.
Oswald, Nevile C.: Recent Trends in Chronic Bronchitis. London, Lloyd-Luke, Ltd., 1958.
Robinson, F. N.: Nursing care of the patient with pulmonary emphysema. Am. J. Nursing, 63:92-96, 1963.
Shafer, K. N., Sawyer, J. R., McCluskey, A. M., and Beck, E. L.: Medical-Surgical Nursing. 3rd Ed. St. Louis, Mo., C. V. Mosby Co., 1964.
Stuart-Harris, C. H.: Chronic Bronchitis, Emphysema and Cor-Pulmonale. Bristol, England, John Wright and Sons, Ltd., 1957.
Williams, M. H.: Pulmonary emphysema, Am. J. Nursing, 63:88-91, 1963.

1186 Hartford Turnpike
North Haven, Connecticut

The Nurse and the Patient with Peripheral Vascular Disease

by AUDREY J. FULCHER, M.A.*

Disorders of the vascular system have long been recognized as devastating threats to the health of mankind. Egyptian mummies show evidence of vascular problems, Hippocrates described clot formation, and one hundred years ago Virchow discovered that portions of the clot could break off and be carried through the blood stream from the point of origin to other parts of the body.

Despite centuries of investigation, vascular diseases continue to be a major health problem. Although great strides have been made in the treatment of these diseases throughout the years, up to the present day more people are disabled by and die from vascular diseases than from diseases of any other origin. The disorders are better understood than ever before, and new treatments have been introduced from time to time, but means of prevention and cure still elude researchers.

Because vascular diseases are so widespread, the nurse will frequently encounter people with these problems who will require her care and guidance. In order to provide skilled, intelligent care to those who are afflicted, and to supply health teaching and guidance in an attempt to prevent subsequent complications, the nurse not only must be familiar with the underlying causes of these diseases, the treatment, and routine nursing care; she must above all understand the patient himself.

ETIOLOGY AND SYMPTOMS

All tissues of the body require circulating blood to supply their metabolic needs, to remove their waste products, and to maintain a relatively stable temperature. Adequate blood supply is vital if tissues are to remain healthy and alive. If the blood supply to a part is reduced for any reason, the part eventually dies.

---

* Instructor, University of Connecticut School of Nursing, Storrs.

When disturbances of blood flow occur, they are likely to be manifested early at the periphery of the vascular bed. Peripheral vessels, especially those of the fingers and toes, are severely affected not only because they are most distal from the heart, but also because they are most likely to be subjected to extremes of temperature and to trauma.

DIMINISHED ARTERIAL SUPPLY

Diminution of arterial blood flow may be the result of a number of causes. Action of the sympathetic nervous system produces constriction of the peripheral vessels and thus limits the blood supply to the extremities even though the vessels are intact. Inflammatory reactions caused by trauma or certain disease organisms may cause swelling of the lining of the vessel and so impede the flow of the lifegiving blood. Or the caliber of the vessel may be altered by the presence of a blood clot or thrombus. Infrequently, distant lesions, tumors, or overgrowth of bone may cause pressure on blood vessels and thus inhibit the supply to the periphery.

Regardless of the underlying cause, all patients with decreased arterial blood flow will exhibit the same symptoms. Relief of these symptoms is afforded only if the underlying cause can be removed.

Symptoms. Ischemia (from the Greek *ischein*, to hold back, and *haima*, blood) is the term used to describe local areas of anemia caused by decreased blood supply. Symptoms of ischemia are coldness of the part, cyanosis or pallor of the skin, cramplike muscle pain, trophic changes in the skin, diminished pulsation of the arteries and, eventually, ulceration and gangrene. Severity of the symptoms depends upon how much tissue is involved and the duration of the constriction.

DISTURBANCES OF VENOUS RETURN

Disturbances of peripheral venous circulation are the result of forces that slow or occlude the venous return. The cause may be from inside the vessel, as in inflammations of the wall of the vein or changes in the composition of the blood; or from distant external causes that prevent proper emptying of the venous flow and so cause stagnation of blood. Any condition that causes stagnation or stasis of blood increases the clot-forming factors of the body. Clot formation or thrombosis causes further restriction of the venous return, and since waste products of metabolism cannot be removed, subsequent death of the tissues of the area occurs.

Symptoms. Symptoms of impaired venous flow include swelling of the area, warm skin, normal arterial pulses, deep red, mottled or

Conditions Causing Reduced Arterial Supply

Disease	Predisposing factors
Buerger's disease or thromboangiitis obliterans	Unknown; suspect infection or activity of some toxic agent
Arteriosclerosis (atherosclerosis)	Diabetes, hypertension, disturbances of lipid metabolism, especially cholesterol
Arterial embolism	Heart disease—atrial fibrillation, vascular lesions, bacterial endocarditis, coronary occlusion, venous thrombosis
Arteritis	Systemic infections—syphilis, pneumonia, typhus fever, typhoid fever, influenza, septicemia, scarlet fever, cholera
Constant constriction of peripheral vessels	Pathologic overactivity of sympathetic nervous system
Spasmodic cyanosis of the fingers	Spondylitis, cervical rib
Frostbite	Exposure to cold

cyanotic skin, dull aching pain and, eventually, ulceration and gangrene. One of the most dangerous elements of thrombosis is the possibility of part of the clot (embolus) breaking off and traveling to a vital center. Pulmonary, coronary, and cerebral emboli are likely to cause sudden and dramatic changes often resulting in death.

If the nurse is aware of the underlying cause of the symptoms

Conditions Causing Decreased Venous Flow.

Disease	Predisposing Factors
Varicose veins	Familial defects of valves, pregnancy, abdominal tumors, ascites
Phlebothrombosis (noninflammatory clot formation)	Heart disease, obesity, varicosities, trauma, surgery, debility, polycythemia, certain anemias
Thrombophlebitis (inflammatory clot formation)	Local injury to endothelium by stretching or trauma, chemical irritation, infection, esp. pneumonia, influenza, typhoid fever. Prolonged bed rest during infections

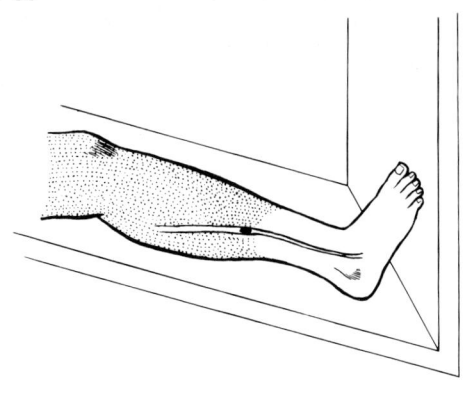

Figure 1. Diagrammatic depiction of area affected by decreased arterial supply to extremity.

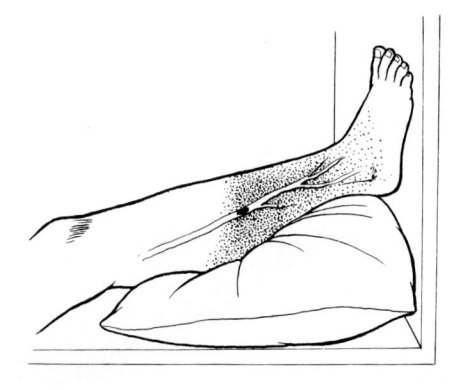

Figure 2. Diagrammatic illustration showing area affected by decreased venous flow.

presented by her patient, she will be prepared to understand the rationale of the treatment prescribed and to provide intelligent care. Success of the treatment will depend upon the ability to remove or lessen the underlying cause, care of the existing damage, and prevention of further injury. Success depends upon the skill of the doctor, the understanding of the nurse, and the cooperation of both the patient and his family.

The accompanying tabulations are presented as a means of recalling to the nurse the conditions that involve arteries or veins.

PATIENTS WITH PERIPHERAL VASCULAR DISEASE

Mr. Aaron Goldberg sat in room 422 with the lights out. Visiting hours had just ended, Miriam and Marvin were on their way home, and he wanted to be alone for awhile. Gosh, how his leg pained; he felt his right foot and it was cold and lifeless. It was better here in the dark because he hated to see how white it looked. In all of his

56 years he had never been so scared. He had never been sick a day in his life. Sure he had those cramps in his foot a couple of years back, but the arch supports seemed to help. The business had really begun to flourish, but he had to keep after those salesmen; who could bother with a few cramps? But now all of a sudden—bed rest —possible gangrene—don't they have to amputate for gangrene? Nine more years to retirement to the lot in Florida and Marvin with two more years of medical school. Gosh, how that foot pains. Pretty soon that nurse—what's her name?—Miss Jones will be in to feel that foot again. Better have another cigarette.

During visiting hours Miss Jones had read Mr. Goldberg's chart. Thromboangiitis obliterans with impending gangrene. Treatment: bed rest, elevate head of bed on 8 inch shock blocks, Buerger's exercises t.i.d., check pedal pulse q. 2 h., phenobarbital gr. 1/2 t.i.d., Demerol 50 mg. I.M. p.r.n. for pain, Priscoline 50 mg. q.i.d., foot cradle—that seems to cover the medical regimen all right. Head of the bed elevated to encourage circulation to the feet, bed rest and foot cradle to limit chances of pressure or trauma to his foot, check pedal pulse to evaluate any change in circulation, phenobarbital to allay apprehension, Demerol for pain, and Priscoline to dilate the blood vessels. Let's see, how do Buerger's exercises go? Oh, yes, legs up two minutes, down two minutes, and flat two minutes; they really help to stimulate circulation. I wonder if they plan for Mr. Goldberg to have a sympathectomy. Actually, I think that the preferred plan is to wait to see how he responds to this medical regimen. These major operations are not necessary when the condition responds well to medical care. I just saw his wife leave—I'll go in now and see if I can make him comfortable for the night.

"If you don't need the big light, Miss Jones, why don't you just use the little one on the dresser? The big one hurts my eyes."

"I'd like to look at your foot when I check your pulse. Does it bother you to look at it?"

"Yes, it scares me to death, it's so white. Do you think it will ever get better?"

"I can understand your concern. This all must have been very sudden for you. I would like very much to help you to get better. The treatment that Dr. White has prescribed has been proved to be quite successful. The exercises and the medications will help to improve your circulation."

"Maybe I should have come into the hospital sooner."

"That is difficult to say. Many times it is impossible to anticipate these problems. Now that you know that you have circulatory problems you can use some caution. I'll be here in the morning and we can talk about some of the precautions you might take when you go home. The pulse in your foot seems a little stronger tonight. I'll turn out the big light now. You can do your exercises with the little one on."

"You know, Miss Jones, leaning the pillows on the cradle like that makes a nice support for my legs. I can just put them right up there without any special equipment. I would rather have them down, but the pillows help a lot. Say, if the doctor wants me to exercise why doesn't he let me walk around?"

"When you walk around, your feet have to carry the weight of your body, which causes a great deal of pressure on them; then, too, you might bump them and embarrass the circulation a little more. These exercises can stimulate the circulation without any pressure or chance of bumping them. There, that's two minutes. Now, I will take the cradle and pillows away and you can put your legs flat on the bed."

"Good, then when I sit up I'll have a cigarette. This foot sure has made me nervous."

"Do you know, Mr. Goldberg, that smoking constricts the blood vessels and limits the circulation to your feet? The cigarettes have just the opposite effect from those white pills you are taking. The pills help to dilate the blood vessels and improve your circulation, while the cigarettes constrict the vessels and limit the circulation."

"I have been smoking since I was 19 years old, you know. I like to have a cigarette when I get nervous."

"Why don't you try to cut down anyway? Maybe you could try to alternate the cigarettes with those sour balls your wife brought you. Have a sour ball for every other cigarette. If you can cut down on your smoking, I think that you will find that your foot will get better much faster."

"I guess I can try. I really do want that foot to get better fast. Can I sit up now—and have a sour ball? Somehow it's not the same though."

"When you are sitting on the edge of the bed like that, push out a little so that your knees do not touch the mattress. That's the way, no pressure on the back of the knees. Now rest your feet on the chair. Why don't you take your pills now while you are sitting up?"

"My foot really feels better when it is down like this. May I stay here for awhile?"

"Yes, why don't you sit there for a few more minutes? I will put this pillow at your back. Meanwhile, I will prepare a medication for you that will help you get a good night's sleep. Tomorrow we can talk more about what you can do to improve your circulation when you get home."

"Thank you, Miss Jones, I think I understand things a little better now."

There now, the Demerol really helped Mr. Goldberg; he went to sleep in half an hour. It really is better to give an analgesic before the pain becomes unbearably severe; it does not have so much to overcome that way. As his circulation improves and the pain lessens, he will not need the medication so often; thus, fear of addiction should not be a great problem. Now, I will just make some notes in the nursing care plan so that we can emphasize future preventive measures to Mr. G. while he is here. We can do them a little at a time as he begins to feel better. Right now his main concern is with the cold, white foot and the pain.

Let's see—preventive measures: (1) Limit smoking; stop if possible. (2) Keep feet warm; avoid extremes of heat or cold, wear woollen socks. (3) Avoid pressure on feet; wear proper fitting shoes. (4) Exercise—walk, not stand; continue Buerger's exercises. (5) Avoid trauma; no bare feet. (6) Avoid infection. Soak feet in warm water every night; dry thoroughly, especially between toes, apply lanolin. (7) Don't cross knees when sitting or cross feet when in bed. (8) Keep covers loose at foot of bed. (9) Drink 8 to 10 glasses of water every day. (10) Continue to visit doctor; take medications he prescribes. There, we can approach these one at a time. Tomorrow when Mrs. Goldberg comes in we can begin to talk together. She will want to know all these preventive measures, too. Now it is time to see Mrs. Johnson.

✷   ✷   ✷

Next door in room 423, Annie Johnson lay still in bed. She had just decided that she had to go home. All this fuss for a little pain in the calf of her leg! Why, last month I had pains in my legs that were no worse than this. Last month, how much had happened! First, Timmy was born, my third baby though first boy; then, just $3\,^{1}/_{2}$ weeks later, the gallbladder operation, and now this. How sudden this had been! My varicose veins always did ache a little, but the elastic stockings that the nurse gave me helped ease that before the operation and I have been wearing them ever since. I didn't notice that tender spot on my leg until yesterday. It did feel hot when I tried to wash my leg. Looked red, too. And now the doctor says it is a clot. The warm soaks make it feel better but once I get up and walk around, the pain will disappear. My legs have ached before. I am not going to take that needle tonight either.

Miss Jones was in the medicine room preparing the heparin for Mrs. Johnson while the saline solution was heating for her soaks.

Heparin 100 mg. I.M. every 12 hours. Let's see now, heparin is the quick-acting anticoagulant. It begins to take effect almost immediately following injection, neutralizes the prothrombin in the blood as I remember. The advantage of this anticoagulant is not only its instantaneous action, but also the fact that the duration of its action is relatively short. This short time of action provides a safety factor in case the prothrombin time falls too rapidly and bleeding occurs. Then just stop the drug—no residual action. Dicumarol is an effective anticoagulant, too. The greatest advantage of Dicumarol is that it is given by mouth. It takes a longer time to act; however, it inhibits production of prothrombin in the liver. It is also difficult to determine the degree of its activity or how long it will last. Mrs. Johnson has only heparin ordered, but often, the two are ordered together: heparin for the instant, short-lasting effects and Dicumarol for the more long-lasting action. The order for the daily prothrombin time has gone to the laboratory. Too bad this happened to Mrs. Johnson—three small children at home—fortunate that her mother can stay to care for them.

"Hello again, Mrs. Johnson. Your soaks must be cooling off now; I would like to reapply them."

"No, Miss Jones, I have decided that I do not need the soaks. I am going home in the morning. My leg feels much better. I am not going to take that needle either. I never did like needles."

"But, Mrs. Johnson, this medication will help you. It will help to make your leg better sooner."

"My leg is better now. I do not need any further treatment. Tomorrow, I will go home. Please call my husband now; he will come for me before he goes to work in the morning."

"Does the needle hurt that much, Mrs. Johnson?"

"The needle doesn't hurt but I do not need the medication now. I will be home tomorrow."

"You must be anxious to get back to your children, too, Mrs. Johnson. Your little one is only a month old, isn't he?"

"Yes, I only had one week at home with him."

"I can understand that you must be concerned about the children, but isn't your mother going to stay with them while you are here?"

"Yes, my mother is there but the children make her nervous. I really cannot stay here."

"Have you been able to talk your mother this week, Mrs. Johnson?"

"No, she stays with the children while my husband comes in."

"Mrs. Johnson, would you like to come with me while I call your home?"

"But the doctor told me to stay in bed."

"I can get a wheel chair and you can ride out to the phone."
Fifteen minutes later:
"You know, Miss Jones, my mother learned how to make Fluffernutters today? Cindy told her where the peanut butter and marshmallow are. And Timmy is taking his bottle just fine. Mom says it is just like old times. She isn't nervous now. Maybe I can stay a few more days. The soaks do make my leg feel better and I really don't mind that needle."

SUMMARY

Disturbances of blood distribution to the peripheral vascular system present symptoms of impaired tissue metabolism and eventually death of the part. New medications and surgical procedures have prolonged the life of many victims, but the cause and cure continue to elude investigators.

Many men with vascular disturbances have used tobacco for years and find it difficult, if not impossible, to break the habit. Constant insistence that the patient "quit smoking" adds to his frustration and anxiety.

Long separation from family and job responsibilities will often cause resistance to treatment. A mother will frequently be more concerned with the welfare of her family than with her own care.

Although nursing care of patients with vascular disease is not complicated, it does involve the whole person. Understanding of the disease and the medical regimen is essential to nursing care. Understanding of the individual is even more vital. Fear of painful treatments or permanent disability causes resistance to care. Exercises, drugs, surgery, soaks, and sedation support life of the tissues, but it is the understanding of the patient as a person that supplies life to the individual.

ACKNOWLEDGMENT

Illustrations for this paper were modified from original drawings by Elaine C. Raymond, M.A.

61 Davis Road
East Hartford, Connecticut

The Nurse's Role in Preventing Circulatory Complications in the Patient with a Fractured Hip

by IMMACULATA M. ALBA, M.A.,*
and JANICE PAPEIKA

It has become increasingly apparent that even in this scientific day and age, nursing intervention in the areas of prevention of illness and rehabilitation still has not become an integral part of the nursing care plan. The concern we feel regarding this lack of intervention on the part of the nurse has been one of the reasons for writing this paper.

When a person is immobilized for any length of time, as with a fractured hip, a process begins, the outcome of which the nurse can to a certain extent predict and control. Nursing care becomes dynamic when the nurse makes meaningful and knowledgeable intervention to restore the patient to his former state of health. Static nursing care enhances the stasis to which the patient is already predisposed. It is the objective of this paper to suggest nursing care measures designed to prevent stasis and its resulting complications. Keeping in mind that stasis affects all body systems, the complications of the circulatory system will be emphasized here, and since most patients with fractured hips are elderly, the particular needs of this age group will be taken into account.

Because the nurse may be caring for a patient at any time during his recovery, it is important to institute the most effective preventive measures appropriate to the point where she begins. For example, the nurse caring for the patient in the immediate postoperative phase has responsibilities that may vary somewhat from those of the nurse who begins caring for a patient who already has signs and symptoms of complications.

---

* Instructor, University of Connecticut School of Nursing, Storrs.

THE PATHOPHYSIOLOGY OF THROMBUS FORMATION

The chief complication with which we are concerned here is thrombus formation. Preventive nursing care is enhanced when the nurse is aware of the pathophysiologic changes leading to thrombus formation. Newton's first law of motion states,

> "Every body perseveres in its state of rest—unless it is compelled to change that state by forces impressed thereon."

Although Newton was not referring to fracture patients, the point is just as appropriate here. When the body is at rest the metabolic needs are reduced, causing a reduction in all body processes. In the circulatory system, this means that cardiac output is diminished. However, the blood volume does not diminish appreciably, and the venous system, acting as a reservoir, tends to become filled. The middle layer or media of the veins contains less elastic and muscular tissue than that of the arteries, so that the veins collapse when empty and do not retain their shape.

Forces which affect the flow of blood through the vessels may be summed up as follows: (1) shape of the vein; (2) straightness of the vessel; (3) muscular activity; (4) viscosity of the blood; (5) gravity; and (6) changes in the size of the lumen of the vessel.

Contraction of the muscles in the extremities facilitates the forward motion of the blood. Blood tends to flow away from the areas of compression and the valves are arranged so that direction of flow can only be toward the heart. Therefore, each time a person tenses his muscles, blood is moved toward the heart. When a patient is immobilized, the muscle "pump" is not in operation and stasis occurs.

The Influence of Age. Stasis, disease, dehydration, and roughening of the vascular endothelium are conditions which may be found in the elderly—even those without an orthopedic condition—all caused either by microorganisms, surgery, or trauma, and all can cause intravascular clotting. In addition, this kind of patient is likely to have one or more chronic diseases which will further decrease his reserve and place an additional burden on his capacity to adapt. This simply means that his body is less able to cope with situations placing stress on his functional capacity.

Senescence brings about fibrotic changes in the vascular system as in the rest of the body. Fibrotic tissue replaces some of the elastic tissue in the media and causes decreased venous return. The veins become dilated and tortuous and the blood cannot move as fast around these curves.

The Effects of Trauma. Trauma usually precedes a fractured hip and the need for surgical intervention to obtain optimal bone union and alignment carries with it the possibility of infection. These factors may destroy the integrity of the vascular wall. Immobility during this time, both preoperatively and postoperatively, predisposes the patient to stasis.

When the rate of blood flow is slowed, cells tend to leave the center of the blood vessels where they are normally concentrated, and move toward the periphery where they come in contact with the vascular walls. Normally, the intima and platelets are mutually repulsive, each being negatively charged to prevent intravascular clotting. However, a damaged wall loses its charge and attracts platelets. The platelets, adhering to the vessel wall, trigger off the clotting mechanism. Leukocytes and large numbers of platelets gather at the site of adherence. The thrombus at this point is not firmly attached, and can become an *embolus*. Clinical evidence of blood flow disturbance and inflammation usually are not present at this stage but may be anticipated at a somewhat later time.

Within the vessel, part of the thrombus is attached at the point of origin. The remaining portion floats freely within the lumen. It becomes adherent when contact is made with the vessel wall, and thus the lumen becomes obstructed. Vasospasm from irritation further constricts the lumen, flow is impeded, and more coagulation takes place. The involved veins reveal edema, degeneration of smooth muscle fibers, and proliferation of fibroblasts. Because of this fibrotic process the valves become thickened, scarred, and completely functionless. Venous walls become sclerotic and their lumens become tortuous and irregular. Permanent disturbances in the hemodynamics occur.

Causes of Embolization. Theories which may explain the embolization of a thrombus suggest that any sudden increase in venous pressure, such as may accompany coughing, sudden motion, and straining at stool, may cause part of the thrombus to break away from the wall, becoming an embolus. Excessive clot retraction occurring in chronic anemia, which is often present in the elderly, because of longstanding poor nutritional habits, or in anemia following surgery, may also tend to loosen the clot from the vessel walls and permit it to be dislodged by the passing stream of blood.

THE NURSE'S ROLE IN PREVENTION OF THROMBOSIS AND EMBOLUS

It would appear that the nurse must act as the "forces impressed thereon" in Newton's first law if she wishes to change the patient's "state of rest." It will undoubtedly fall to the nurse to plan with the physician those nursing measures that will prevent these complications.

Gluteal and quadriceps setting exercises are valuable supplements to the usual range of motion exercises because they are easy to perform, painless, and can be done without much supervision. Footboard walking is another easy feat for the patient to perform on his own, once it is explained to him. The use of an overhead trapeze or rope attached to the foot of the bed allows the patient to actively exercise the upper extremities and trunk and gives him more independence. The trend toward early ambulation with help can be included as a factor of major importance. Deep breathing exercises, coughing, and turning should still be considered essentials in preventing stasis in the pulmonary vascular bed.

In view of the relative lack of elasticity of the veins and the structure and function of the valves, position plays an important part in venous return. The patient may usually be turned from side to side and the legs may be elevated to promote flow toward the heart. As mentioned earlier, changes in the size of the lumen affect blood flow. When the vessel is compressed, blood cannot flow through readily. The straighter the vessel, the less resistance to flow. Constant flexion of any joint must be avoided since it causes compression and subsequent pooling of blood. Use of the Gatch bed, pillows or rolls under the knees or other positions causing flexion should be approached with caution.

Properly used, elastic stockings provide support for tired, sagging veins. The stockings must be of the correct size and must be removed at least once every 8 hours, so that they do not act as a tourniquet. If edema, mottling of the skin, numbness, tingling, or cold feet occur, the stockings should be removed at once. The patient's subjective signs may be the first clue a nurse has that something is wrong.

Since dehydration increases the viscosity of blood, adequate hydration is necessary to prevent intravascular clotting. Thus the forcing of fluids assumes prime importance and cannot be minimized.

Securing the Patient's Cooperation. Patients having reparative surgery of the hip do not willingly accept turning, no matter how lofty the goals of the nurse. The discomfort of the patient is probably the chief reason meaningful nursing intervention is not undertaken. Even the most knowledgeable and technically competent nurse may often be deterred from doing what she knows to be best—in this case turning and moving the patient to prevent the complications that she knows may begin to appear postoperatively.

Several approaches to this problem that we have found helpful include administering analgesics a half hour before attempting to reposition or exercise the patient, and preparing the patient preoperatively for the exercises and movements that will be expected of him after surgery. Careful, clear explanations before attempting to move him and the provision of sufficient assistance will all be of help in reducing fear and pain. The nurse should also enlist the cooperation of family members to provide the emotional support so necessary during times of stress.

Above all, the nurse must know her patient: she must recognize his limitations; aid him to set goals for himself and allow him to set the limits of his capabilities, and then support him in his attempt to meet these goals.

We strongly maintain that the nurse, who spends more time with the patient than anyone else, is in a far better position to prevent circulatory complications of the fracture patient than any other member of the health team.

REFERENCES

Beland, Irene L., Read, Esther H., Ronan, Jane F., Passos, Joyce, and Martin, Nancy: Clinical Nursing—Pathophysiological and Psychosocial Approaches. New York, The Macmillan Co., 1965.

Beeson, P. B., and McDermott, W., Eds.: Cecil-Loeb Textbook of Medicine. 11th Ed. Philadelphia, W. B. Saunders Co., 1963.

Harrison, T. R.; Principles of Internal Medicine. 4th Ed. Blakiston Division, McGraw-Hill Book Co., 1962.

430 Third Avenue
West Haven, Connecticut 06516

Cerebrovascular Accident: The Role of the Public Health Nurse

by HARRIETT L. WILCOXSON, M.A.*

Of the three major causes of death today in the United States, the least attention, research, and care is given to cerebrovascular accidents. For many years there was a fatalistic attitude toward this condition. Yet the medical and nursing literature of the last decade is increasingly offering hope—hope that much of the suffering and disability can be prevented or delayed for years with the aid of skillful diagnosis and treatment.

The concern of this paper is an account of the magnitude of the problem of cerebrovascular accident, of the status of preventive measures, and the role of the public health nurse in prevention and care.

WHAT DO WE MEAN BY A CEREBROVASCULAR ACCIDENT?

The brain, because of its high energy requirement, demands over a fifth of all the blood pumped from the heart. If circulation to the brain fails as a result of disease of the blood vessels, a cerebrovascular accident (often called a "stroke," and often abbreviated C.V.A.) results.

There are, generally speaking, there main types of cerebrovascular accident:

1. Those due to occlusion by thrombosis of a diseased vessel.
2. Those due to occlusion by a fragment of a clot which becomes dislodged from the heart or the vessels of the neck and plugs a cerebral vessel.
3. Those due to rupture of a cerebral vessel as a result of high blood pressure or an aneurysm.

---

* Assistant Professor, University of Connecticut School of Nursing, Storrs.

THE EXTENT OF THE PROBLEM

Stroke ranks third as an overall cause of death. Although it is thought of essentially as a disease of the aged, it is the fifth most frequent killer of persons under 65, people often in the most productive years of life. It is outranked only by heart disease, cancer, accidents, and suicides for this age group.[9]

At least 2 million people in the United States have suffered a stroke. Eight out of 10 people survive the initial phase and most of them live on for some years, usually in a seriously disabled condition. The economic cost to the nation in 1962 was approximately $1.1 billion.[9]

Given these few simple but startling facts it seems worth while for the public health nurse to ask herself what she can do to help prevent the human misery inherent in these figures.

MEASURES TO HELP PREVENT THIS DISEASE AND LIMIT CRIPPLING

Slowly mounting interest over the past decade has revealed genuine hope for C.V.A. victims. No longer need this condition be considered inevitable and irremediable. There are promising new avenues for research which in time should lead to more effective prevention and rehabilitation.

In the meantime, there are many warning symptoms of cerebrovascular disease which if detected and treated may save the potential victim years of suffering. The medical profession may be able to help the potential C.V.A. patient with antihypertensive drugs, anticoagulants, and/or surgery of the vascular system. It has been shown that early, intensive, modern rehabilitation can restore as many as 80 per cent of stroke survivors to a relatively active and productive life.[9]

THE PUBLIC HEALTH NURSE'S ROLE IN PREVENTION

The nurse needs to understand that most of the distress caused by a cerebrovascular accident can be alleviated by the timely application of preventive or rehabilitative treatment. She should know that a patient who complains of brief attacks of loss of speech, weakness of limbs, staggering, or loss of consciousness should be directed toward medical attention without delay. The nurse needs to know also that those in whom a cerebrovascular accident cannot be prevented can be helped effectively by early and continuous rehabilitation. She should familiarize herself with the medical and rehabilitation facilities available in the community in which she is working and the way in which she fits into the community program.

Every public health nurse has the opportunity during home and conference visits to do case finding provided she is alert to danger symptoms and makes appropriate medical referrals. In many communities that is all she has the opportunity to do. However, in Hartford, Connecticut, a public health nurse is working with a selected group of citizens in a preventive program. This is not a unique program but it was one of the early examples of a community striving to encourage its senior citizens, to function on a level of activity more satisfying to them and to prevent or delay the disabling effects of chronic disease.

As part of an overall interest on the part of various health and welfare agencies in the needs of the geriatric population of the city of Hartford, a demonstration Geriatric Medical Clinic was established at the Charter Oak Terrace Housing Project in February, 1962. This pilot study lasting 10 weeks was sponsored by the Hartford Health Department. A part-time physician was employed who worked in cooperation with the public health nurses and the housing project's tenant advisor.

Charter Oak Terrace is a low income housing project in which approximately 5500 persons live. For this study only those over 65 years of age were considered. There were 226 persons in this age group, and of these 100 were studied. The persons selected for study were chosen because they requested the service or were encouraged to attend by the public health nurse because of overt symptoms. A medical history and a physical examination were completed on all patients, approximately one hour being spent with each individual. Of the 100 patients studied, 64 patients exhibited 98 ailments that required further evaluation and treatment. Twenty-seven of these ailments were cardiovascular in nature. Eighty-eight per cent of the 64 patients with specific needs sought follow-up care. As a result of this it was felt that 56 per cent benefited physically from these services and 50 per cent benefited emotionally.[1]

The success of this demonstration was in large part due to the confidence and trust the patients had in their public health nurse and tenant advisor, who did much work in contacting families and interpreting the program. Particular benefits of the project included the fact that the clinic was brought to the patient, all his complaints were considered in one place by one doctor, and he was treated as an individual with potentially multiple chronic disease, not just as an impersonal list of diseases. He himself, through the housing project's "Over-Sixty Club," participated in requesting and organizing this program. The public health nurse enthusiastically made follow-up visits to ascertain the patient's progress in seeking needed medical attention and she assisted him in carrying out recommendations when needed.

It is not difficult to see the potential of such a program in terms of prevention of human suffering caused by increasingly debilitating chronic disease. It is encouraging to note that the value of this program was recognized and it has been continued by the Department of Health of the City of Hartford.

Other functions of the nurse include working with patients who are overweight and might have a tendency to cardiovascular disease, and discussing diet with patients who have high blood pressure. It is not enough that patients know the basic four food groups: this knowledge does them no good unless the patients and families know what to buy, how to prepare it, and then eat it in quantities commensurate with their needs. The nurse discusses also other aspects of healthful living such as physical and mental activities that provide relaxation from tensions and add zest to living.

In summary, then, the nurse has an important role to play in bridging the gap between the discovery of scientific facts and their application to the public.

TREATMENT OF THE STROKE PATIENT

The nurse might first examine her own feelings about this disease and those afflicted by it. Nurses along with the general public have long believed this to be a disease that caused death in the patient sooner or later, and that if it did not kill, it at least so severely damaged the brain that the patient would no longer be a useful member of society. Lack of dramatic improvement in the patient after extended care is a discouraging factor to many nurses. Also, the personality changes in the patient often make him a very unattractive and unrewarding person to care for. There are several books and articles in current literature that inspire the nurse to greater understanding and compassion for a person afflicted with C.V.A.

Eric Hodgins' book *Episode*[6] tells the story of his cerebrovascular accident and the long, difficult, and tedious road to recovery. It shows us dramatically his reaction to nurses who considered him as a person with desires and interests important to himself. It also shows the reaction of the patient to nurses who tended his physical needs without making any effort to understand him personally, attempting instead to convert him to their pet health or religious theories to which he reacted negatively. It illustrates forcefully his real progress or lack of it toward rehabilitation under each type of care.

Genevieve Smith in her book *Care of the Patient with a Stroke*[10] writes with sympathy and understanding of the severely stricken C.

V.A. patient, who in this case happened to be her husband. Since she is a nurse the information she imports is clear and factual from a nursing point of view, and the reader in addition sees how the tremendous amount of physical and emotional energy expended in the care of the patient can be worth while.

Another facet of the frustrating probelms presented by the C.V.A. patient is the frequently noted inability to communicate. Many nurses have little real appreciation of what this means to a patient. Broadway took this problem as a theme and produced a thrillingly forceful play entitled *The Miracle Worker*.[5] The climax of this absorbing production was the point at which the child, Helen Keller, and the teacher, Annie Sullivan, achieved communication.

THE PATIENT IN HIS HOME SETTING

The nurse starts with the patient at whatever level of progress, or lack of progress, she may find him. She considers the physical aspects of the home setting; she assesses not only the patient's potential but the attitude, strengths, and weaknesses of the family, and from these she makes her nursing diagnosis.

If the patient has been hospitalized there is, hopefully, a detailed medical referral indicating as far as possible the patient's potential for continued improvement as well as a plan of treatment. If the patient is now under the care of his family physician instead of the hospital medical staff, the nurse discusses with the family doctor his plans for treatment of the patient.

The physical aspects of the home must be evaluated in the terms of the patient's needs. Are the doors wide enough to accommodate a wheel chair, if necessary? How many steps are there between the patient's bedroom, the bathroom, and the family living room? Are there door sills, scatter rugs, and highly polished floors that will be of potential danger to the patient? Is the patient's bed of a height that will make the nurse's and family's care of him easy and also make his bed-to-chair transfer relatively safe?

The nurse also needs to judge the emotional climate of a home. There are homes where the patients are wanted and needed and the families will do all in their power under guidance to help the patient. There are homes where the family members find it difficult to assume a firmness that is often needed with the C.V.A. patient. There are homes where the sons and daughters may feel a duty to care for a formerly domineering parent, but would rather keep him in the back room or upstairs so that he interferes only at a minimum with family activities. There are also homes in which the patient has waited hand and foot on the children and now thinks it is time for the family to wait on him (or more often her). There are normally varying degrees of skill exhibited by members of the family in caring for an ill person. There are families that pull together at times of illness and there are families that break apart under such stress. A nurse must assess all these factors and more while trying to arrive at a nursing care plan for the patient.

The nurse not only needs to know what care the patient has received previously but also what kind of a person he was before he was stricken, what his likes and dislikes were, his personality traits and interests. The disease may have resulted in a personality reversal. In many instances this knowledge helps in understanding the patient and gaining his cooperation in the struggle of rehabilitation. If the nurse knows "what makes him tick," it is often possible to find out what will move him to take and to continue positive steps in the long struggle back to a useful life. This information may also make it possible for the nurse to feel a liking and warmth that the patient's post-stoke personality may inhibit. If a nurse is to establish a meaningful relationship with the patient it is helpful for her to let him know she likes him, and the best way to show liking is to feel it. Words without feeling are empty but feeling can often be conveyed without words.

PHYSICAL CARE

In the physical care of the patient the nurse has a number of concerns. In the prevention of *deformities,* the nurse should be aware that getting the bed patient into the prone position for one-half hour several times a day is an aid in preventing contractures; that the gravity pull of the paralyzed arm puts a strain on the shoulder of the affected side which can cause considerable pain, and which in turn interferes with rehabilitation; that changing the patient's position hourly is helpful in preventing decubiti; that it is often easier for the patient to use a commode than a bedpan; that range of motion exercises must be done for the nonaffected side as well as the paralyzed side; and that the patient should be expected to carry out only as many of these activities as he can accomplish without undue fatigue. In these responsibilities the nurse has the aid and guidance of the physical therapist as well as many excellent references on the subject.

When *aphasia* is present a speech evaluation is necessary to ascertain the kind and degree of damage. Aphasia may be manifested in any or all language modalities: speaking, reading, writing, calculation, or auditory comprehension. It is well for the nurse to know the aims and the methods of the speech therapist so that all who have contact with a patient may have a consistent approach. If the public health nurse is working in a community where speech therapy is not available it may help her to remember that a stroke patient often learns to speak over again much as he did originally; that is, he first learns nouns, then verbs, then adjectives, adverbs, prepositions, and finally more complex sentence structure. The nurse should always keep in mind that intelligible speech, not perfect speech, is the end toward which to strive.

Diet is another consideration. Often after a stroke a patient may be placed on a low calorie, low sodium, or low cholesterol diet. Not only is he scared and confused by his physical condition but he is trying to come to terms with overwhelming stress. In addition, he is being served food that is not to his liking. When the nurse works with the family concerning the patient's diet she starts with the things the patient has always liked, and using these as a nucleus she can often work out a compromise that is acceptable to the patient. For example, if sodium intake is reduced the patient has to be encouraged to use other seasonings. This takes imaginative cooking on the part of the family. A nutrition consultant can give the nurse and the family many practical suggestions within the limits set up by medical orders, the family's ability to provide, and the patient's likes and dislikes.

In some patients *incontinence* is a problem. Sometimes it is due to severe brain damage but it may also be due to the patient's inability to communicate. In any event, efforts to retrain are helpful for the patient and his family both from a physical and an emotional standpoint.

SUPLEMENTARY SERVICES

The public health nurse needs to be aware of the many facilities in the community that might offer further assistance to a patient with a cerebrovascular accident. He has in many instances already been a patient in the general hospital and has used its department of physical medicine. In some instances he may return to the hospital for outpatient rehabilitation services. However, he may be transferred to the local Easter Seal agency. Many times he needs the help of other disciplines and the community may offer these in a formal Home Care Program. Among the services included in a home care program that are of help to the patient with a stroke are: medical social work, physical therapy, occupational therapy, speech therapy, homemaker services, loan closets, and meals on wheels. These are all services used to supplement the work of the family and the public health nurse.

MOTIVATION

The nurse has to be concerned with the patient's motivation. As a rule the aged hemiplegic patient is not motivated, in the common sense of the word. He seldom actually expresses the desire to be rehabilitated and he presents no problems of vocational rehabilitation, since he usually was not gainfully employed at the time of his illness.

When a patient is stricken with a cerebrovascular accident his reactions include mental changes due to brain damage, and often a depressive reaction to the threat of deterioration and death, and to physical incapacity. It is helpful to the nurse to know of some things that a patient formerly enjoyed that may aid in getting him to work toward his rehabilitation. This brings to mind a situation where the initial insult was not severe and the motivation was high:

> Mr. and Mrs. C. were a couple in their seventies who had been happily married for 48 years. They were still enjoying life to the fullest when Mr. C. was stricken. He had a left-sided paralysis but his doctor felt that his prognosis for recovery from this episode was good. The public health nurse was given orders relative to exercise, diet, and general activity. The patient and his wife were so eager to do what was recommended that they would have worked at it for 26 hours a day, were the hours available. They stated to the nurse they had enjoyed going out in their automobile, visiting friends, dining out, and they aimed to do it again. They did.

Another brief illustration shows how a septuagenarian living alone met the situation of a cerebrovascular accident.

> Miss A., 78 years old, lived in a large old home that had been in the family for a hundred years. She had numerous chronic ailments including generalized arteriosclerosis, arteriosclerotic heart disease, and left hemiplegia. She was hospitalized in a rehabilitation hospital following her stay in a general hospital. She was placed on the local Home Care Program when discharged from the rehabilitation hospital. She became able to walk although she had no visible use of her left hand. She maintained herself in her own home with the aid of a housekeeper companion and the public health nurse. She had no close family but her friends helped to keep her mind active by encouraging her to pursue her hobby of genealogy. She had the books and they gave her problems that kept her busy in "research." The Visiting Nurse Association gave her supportive care which helped to maintain her in her own home where she could live a happier and more active life until such time as her variety of chronic ailments totally disabled her.

The younger hemiplegia patient has another type of attitude or motivation for recovery. This case situation illustrates one type of motivation sometimes found.

> Mr. B. was 52 years old and a widower with two children ages 19 and 21 at the time he became ill. He had a right hemiplegia which, though not too severe, left him with a noticeable disability of his right hand. When he left the hospital the doctor did not encourage him with any hope for return of usefulness in his hand. However, exercises for the affected parts were given and the public health nurse was asked to help. The nurse had never seen a

patient more determined to recover. He desired to return to work and not to be a burden to his children. Also, he added, he was going to write a letter to his doctor and he was going to write it with his right hand. Within seven months he was able to do this and was also contemplating a return to work in the near future.

SUMMARY

Cerebrovascular accident is an important health problem—the third greatest cause of death in the United States today. Although in the past there has been much less interest in this disease than in heart disease and cancer on the part of public health and medical authorities, during the last decade there has been rising interest in and hope for the future of patients threatened with this disease.

The public health nurse has an important role to play in case finding, promotion of prevention programs, education of the public, and assisting in research, as these activities relate to cerebrovascular disease.

The city of Hartford, Connecticut, has a limited but ongoing geriatric clinic program which is helping to detect patients who might well be potential victims of a stroke, and who through this program are referred for definitive diagnosis and treatment. This is an initial step in the right direction in the battle for prevention, and one that might well be taken by other communities and agencies.

For those who have been stricken by illness the public health nurse is on hand to help the family understand and adjust to the member who has had the stroke. She works with the family and patients in the areas of diet, therapeutic bathing, exercise, and mental health. She interprets the services of other community agencies and works with them as needed. She especially finds the services of the physical therapist, occupational therapist, speech therapist, mental health consultant, and nutrition consultant invaluable in her efforts to give comprehensive care to patient and family.

The field of nursing is expanding in an exciting way, offering unlimited horizons to the public health nurse in the prevention of the disease and in the care of the patient with a cerebrovascular accident.

REFERENCES

1. Blanchard, B. M., and Smith, K. M.: A Study of 100 Patients as Seen in the Geriatric Clinic at Charter Oak Terrace Housing Project, Hartford, Conn., February 1962 to February 1963. Unpubished data from Hartford Health Department, Hartford, Conn., May 1963.
2. Buchanan, J. J.: Observations on 1500 patients: rapid mobilization of patients following cerebrovascular accident. South. M. J., 52:1149–1150, 1959.

3. Buck, M.: Adjustments during recovery from stroke. Am. J. Nursing, 64:92–95, 1964.
4. Eisenberg, H., Morrison, J. T., Sullivan, P., and Foote, F. M.: Cerebrovascular accidents, incidence and survival rates in a defined population, Middlesex County, Connecticut. J.A.M.A., 189:883–889, 1964.
5. Gibson, William: The Miracle Worker. New York, Atheneum, 1956.
6. Hodgins, Eric: Episode. New York, Atheneum, 1964.
7. Leone, L. P.: Attack on heart disease, cancer and stroke—is nursing ready? Am. J. Nursing, 65:68–72, 1965.
8. Peszczynski, M.: The rehabilitation potential of the late adult hemiplegic. Am. J. Nursing, 63:111–114, 1963.
9. President's Commission on Heart Disease, Cancer and Stroke: Report to the President—A National Program to Conquer Heart Disease, Cancer and Stroke. Washington, D.C., U.S. Government Printing Office. Vol. I, Dec. 1964. Vol. II, Feb. 1965.
10. Smith, G. W.: Care of the Patient with a Stroke. New York, Springer Publishing Company, 1959.
11. Whitehouse, F. A.: Stroke: some psychosocial problems it causes. Am. J. Nursing, 63:81–87, 1963.
12. Wright, I. S.: A profile of cerebral vascular accidents today. G P, 19:117–127, 1959.
13. Wright, I. S.: Strokes—diagnosis and modern treatment: I. Diagnosis. Mod. Concepts Cardiovas. Dis. 28:519–523, 1959. II. Mod. Concepts Cardiovas. Dis., 34:35–39, 1965.

40 Woodland Street
Hartford, Connecticut 06105

Symposium on The Nurse and the Ill Child

FOREWORD

Every nurse, regardless of her specialty, will inevitably come in contact with children, particularly today when the concept of family centered nursing has become an essential part of the comprehensive care of patients. Therefore, a symposium on the nurse and the ill child has been selected to appear in the first issue of the Nursing Clinics of North America.

The symposium represents a selective series of articles dealing with trends in pediatric nursing as well as current concepts and techniques. We must understand what is happening today, but we must also prepare ourselves for changes that will occur in the near future. Our role as pediatric nurses, whether it be as staff nurses, administrators or educators, is a changing one. This symposium on the nurse and the ill child is designed to help the pediatric nurse function more effectively today, as well as to gain insight into tomorrow's world of nursing practice.

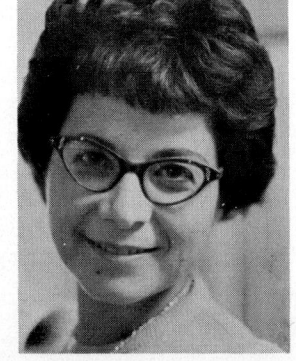

Since the articles are designed to offer depth of understanding of concepts of comprehensive pediatric nursing, an analysis of three essential components of comprehensive nursing may be in order here. Comprehensive nursing encompasses all activities of the nurse that help to attain the goal of meeting individual needs of patients. These include:

1. A philosophy, which is the motivating force.
2. A purpose, with its guiding objectives.
3. An implementation process, with the patient's needs as the core of all activity.

The discussions of "Pediatric Rooming-In" and "The Nurse's Role in Fetal Medicine" focus on changes in the role of the nurse as it is affected by the changing philosophy of pediatric therapy.

"Nursing in the New Pediatrics" offers insight into the nursing world of tomorrow, with its changing forces and new demands that necessitate clear identification of nursing objectives. A paper concerning the exploration of the nurse's own emotions in terms of their effect on objectives and standards of practice is also presented.

Aspects of the implementation process are presented in papers concerning new machinery and changing environments that have placed increasing demands upon nursing in relation to the attainment of specific therapeutic goals in the hospital as well as in the community.

A paper concerning an age-old but essential responsibility of a pediatric nurse—the administration of medications to infants and children—is presented in terms of the physiological bases for drug administration. This paper demonstrates clearly how the basic fields of anatomy and physiology form a foundation for some of the physical aspects of nursing care and for sound nursing judgments.

Each paper is presented by a nurse especially knowledgeable within her respective field. The editor and the authors of the articles in this symposium hope that their efforts will contribute new and useful information that will be of practical value for the reader in her profession as a practicing nurse, as well as for inservice education programs across the country.

GLORIA LEIFER, M.A.
Department of Nursing Education
Hunter College of the City of New York

Nursing and the New Pediatrics

by ELEANOR RUDICK, Ed.D.*

"Pediatrics may be defined as child care that encompasses the child as an individual in a family, and includes the care of the child in health and in illness."[1] Gentle colleague, allow us to anticipate your reaction to the apparent ambiguity of the title and the opening quotation. What indeed is "new" about pediatrics as defined thus? Admittedly, the basic belief may not be new to us, but the means by which the philosophical statement becomes operational are changing as the social context in which we practice is changing. Furthermore, as the nature of the practice of pediatrics changes, so, we submit, does the nature of the nursing of children and the preparation therefor.

TRENDS OF THE NEW PEDIATRICS

In what directions is child care moving to warrant the use of the term "new pediatrics"? The new pediatrics can be characterized by increased emphasis on the inclusion of behavioral and social aspects of care; by movement toward ambulatory care; by movement toward multiprofessional care, requiring coordination; by movement into the community and into the household; by movement toward more concern with prenatal care; and by a trend toward the recognition of the particular needs of adolescents.

SOCIAL-BEHAVIORAL ORIENTATION

We have moved from the central nursery concept of infant care to a concept of care that is family centered. We are learning more about growing and developing children and, as we use our knowledge, we appreciate the need of all children for a family; we recognize that a child without a family is not a normal child. We are aware of the

---

* Assistant Professor, Department of Nursing Education, Teachers College, Columbia University, New York.

dangers of separation and have begun to open hospitals to parents, not because it is their "right," but because they are as necessary to a child's care as are drugs.

We are beginning to realize that with rapid change and increasing complexity of the social order old standards no longer apply. The resulting instability is causing changes in family structure and relationships and as a result parents are seeking assistance with child rearing. As levels of sophistication improve, parents tend to seek that assistance of professionals.

We are learning more about socially derived illness and the effects of social pathology on families and growing children. This has meant, not only the use of the skills of the behavioral and social sciences in basic preparation and in practice, but the introduction of the psychologist and social worker to the child care setting.

AMBULATORY CARE AND THE MULTIPROFESSIONAL TEAM

Childhood morbidity and mortality patterns have changed dramatically in the last fifty years; much disease that was epidemic is now preventable. Children are now living who in earlier days would not have survived premature birth, infection or congenital malformation. The very definition of health has been broadened to include social and emotional well being as well as physical well being. If then we accept the interrelatedness of social, psychological and physical factors in the promotion of health, are we not required to weigh the effect on practice and on facilities for care as well? If, for instance, we believe that children need families, that separation can be traumatic, are we not required to reevaluate some of our more traditional practices? The cost of hospitalization, and the sheer numbers of children, will undoubtedly be influential to this end as well.

Furthermore, as we continue to broaden our concept of care and increase the numbers of "caring professionals," will not our changing philosophy have to be reflected in the type of facilities in which health supervision and treatment are offered? The very bases on which it is decided to hospitalize a child are changing; the degree of illness is but one. We have learned to consider the ability of the mother to cope with the ill child within the family setting as one important criterion when there is a question of the need for hospitalization.

There is change not only in the criteria for hospitalization of children, but also in the very nature of hospital services. In discussing trends in hospital care, Wallace[2] states that there has been a "lessening demand for inpatient hospital care of children with certain diagnoses" and "there has been a concomitant increase in the need for outpatient hospital facilities for children. The concept of the role of the hospital in the community has been broadened.... As new knowledge is being developed in the care of certain types of children (those with hearing impairment, epilepsy, etc.), new services are being developed for them on a predominantly outpatient basis. Hospital outpatient departments are taking on other types of services as well; examples of this are provision of services for health supervision of children, for adolescents, and for children with mental retardation.

"A trend affecting both inpatient and outpatient hospital services has been the gradually increasing role played by the hospital in the rehabilitation of handicapped children.... Still another trend has been the extension and projection of hospital services into the community."[2]

Our hospitals have reflected the problems that *were*. For the new pediatrics the caring facilities must reflect the problems that *are*. The community oriented ambulatory unit, staffed by the multiprofessional team of pediatrician, psychiatrist and/or psychologist, social worker, professional nurse and nutritionist (with assistance from other medical specialists as needed), represents a way in which children and their families in their communities can be provided with care which reflects our understanding of the interrelated concerns of all who contribute. The various professionals as a team, we submit, can offer a whole which is greater than the sum of its parts.

COMMUNITY ORIENTATION

Traditionally, the needs of hospitalized children have determined what the practice of physicians and nurses would be. However, with the new orientation to the indivisible compound of social, emotional and physical components of health, directions for practice must be derived from the total social context. The caring facilities will reflect their communities' needs. It can be argued that this has always been so, that facilities and practice have always reflected social need. For example, well-baby stations and public health nursing itself grew out of obvious community need.

Our thesis is simply that as society, communities and families change, so do their health needs. Yet the traditional notion of pediatric nursing as the care of sick children persists.

PRENATAL CARE

The purview of pediatrics is being extended into the prenatal period as it is becoming recognized that "the major group of illnesses to be found in the average large children's inpatient service today are conditions that are prenatal in origin."[3] At the same time the problem of responsibility for the fetus and the neonate—whether obstetric or pediatric—is being resolved for us. They are the individual responsibility of neither. Rather, they are the responsibility of both.

In line with the increasing knowledge of the importance of emotional factors to health, we are more and more concerned with the emotions of the pregnant woman, recognizing that unresolved difficulties from her own childhood, if they exist, can mar good beginning relationships for the new member of the family.

EXTENDED ADOLESCENCE

The period of adolescence in our society (at least in the social and economic sense) is being extended to about 25 years of age for boys and about 21 years of age for girls. The educational requirements of our highly complex technology are forcing a longer and longer period of economic dependence. At the same time, the shift from a predominantly agrarian to a predominantly urban society has changed family structure and depersonalized neighborhoods, undermining these sources of security for this group of older children for whom support and security are of vital importance.

This protracted period of adolescence, with all its emotional, social and physical changes, requires health services which are neither for the child nor for the adult but are specific to its needs.

WHAT DO THESE CHANGES MEAN FOR THE NURSE?

If, as suggested earlier, nursing is to be as responsive to community health needs as are other social welfare services, let us explore the possible effects of changing pediatric practices on the nursing of children.

THE NURSE AND THE TEAM

The broadened scope of pediatric concern and the evolution of team practice require, we believe, that the professional nurse be prepared to function as a member of this multiprofessional group in a colleague relationship. Furthermore, just as the pediatrician is logically the team leader, the professional nurse is logically the team coordinator. Logically, we say, because preparation for nursing includes something of each of the areas which the other team members represent. "She is," as Caplan[4] states, "a general practitioner among the many specialists who operate in maternal and child care—obstetricians, pediatricians, nutritionists, psychiatrists, psychologists and social workers; she must know something of each of these specialties, and yet she is not competent to operate independently in any of them."

THE NURSE AND THE WELL CHILD

Interestingly, we accept the fact that the pediatrician supervises the growing and developing child, but apparently find it difficult to accept the idea that the professional nurses working with children have anything to contribute in this area. However, as part of the changing scene in pediatrics, the professional nurse can be expected to assume increasing responsibility for much of the supervision of the well child, with the pediatrician in a consultant capacity. Care then is continuous as the child grows and as he—well or sick—returns to see "his nurse" and "his doctor." The continuity provides opportunity for ongoing assessment of growth, development and parent-child relationships. The nurse-child relationships that are formed as a result of such continued association enable the nurse to offer anticipatory guidance based on what she observes the child doing and what she knows about physical and emotional development.

THE NURSE IN THE HOME

The professional nurse, we believe, should be able to extend health service from the ambulatory care unit to the home. On the basis of her observations, and in consultation with her colleagues, she should be able to determine need for home visits and make them herself. Often, the doctor's office (irrespective of location or type of practice) is not the ideal situation in which to assess a child's behavior, and if more needs to be known in order to reach intelligent conclusions, then observation of the youngster at home or at school may provide such opportunity. That much of this kind of observation is provided through efficient referral is, of course, quite true; that "continuity of care" is a concern today is quite true. But we must move from a concept of agency to agency continuity to one of person to person continuity within the multiprofessional setting.

THE NURSE'S ROLE IN GENERAL

Briefly, then, we believe that the following activities constitute the broadening role of the professional nurse working with children in any setting:
1. Interviewing mothers and children in order to begin to assess:
   a. Mother-child relationship
   b. Need for anticipatory guidance
2. Working with physicians and other team members in colleague relationship.
3. Observing children with peers and adults in order to begin to assess developmental status—physical, social and emotional.

4. Making judgments about the need for the extension of nursing care outside institutions to home and community and developing the ability to personally extend nursing care from one institution to another or to the home.

Again, gentle colleague, allow us to anticipate your reaction. You may well be saying at this point that the kind of nursing practice proposed here is quite suitable to the care of children on an ambulatory basis, but not to the care of children in hospitals. But, do we not have a responsibility to use our knowledge of growth, development and family life to advantage when youngsters are sick and cannot be cared for at home?

You may also say that we are attempting to do this. We have begun to liberalize visiting hours for parents; some of us encourage rooming in for preschool children (see p. 83); we prepare children for hospitalization, for surgery and other procedures; we encourage "acting out" afterward; we accept the idea that a hospitalized child need not be confined to bed and that he requires room and equipment for play. But can we not move beyond this, especially in the light of the observation "that for some children hospitalization was a constructive experience which seemed to facilitate rather than impair their growth"?[5] We submit that the nursing care of children can no longer be determined by the facility in which it is given, but rather by the needs of the children wherever we work with them.

IMPLICATIONS FOR NURSING EDUCATION

Preparation to function within this broadened context requires, we believe, that learning to nurse be approached in a spirit of inquiry. Together, students and teacher must explore the components of the professional nurse's role, building on what is known and seeking what needs to be known. Each student finds out for herself what activities constitute that role and how her contributions complement those of the other professionals on the team. Rather than seeing the various professional roles sharply defined, she should be encouraged to develop a feeling for the "gray areas" of overlapping and interdependence.

Selected experience, then, instead of being used to carry out procedures or apply theory learned in the classroom, becomes the heart of the matter—the source of problems to be solved. The teacher is responsible for seeing that the "problem grows out of the conditions of the experience being had in the present ... and that it is such that it arouses in the learner an active quest for information and for the production of new ideas."[7] Classes are used to intellectualize experience in a continuous process of reconstruction, the products of which feed back into practice, thereby raising the level of ability of the student. This is not to suggest that the "content" of nursing be neglected, but that content be defined as process rather than static subject matter. In this way, knowledge and understanding themselves become the means for yet further inquiry.

SUMMARY

There are identifiable trends in the pediatric world: toward ambulatory care, multiprofessional care and social-behavioral orientation; into the community, into the household; extending into prenatal care; extending the duration of adolescence.

Our concern is with the effects of all of this on professional nursing, and we believe that it means a broadened role for which the nurse will need preparation.

REFERENCES

1. Solnit, A. J., and Senn, M. J. E.: Teaching comprehensive pediatrics in an outpatient clinic. Pediatrics. 14:547–556, 1954.
2. Wallace, H. M.: Health Services for Mothers and Children. Philadelphia, W. B. Saunders Co., 1962, pp. 255, 256.
3. Lesser, A.: Health of Children of School Age. U.S. Department of Health, Education, and Welfare. Children's Bureau Publication No. 427, 1964.
4. Caplan, G.: An Approach to Community Mental Health. New York, Grune & Stratton, 1961, p. 176.
5. Shore, M. F., et al.: Constructive uses of a hospital experience. Children, 12:3–8, 1965.
6. Dewey, J.: Experience and Education. New York, The Macmillan Company, 1959, p. 97.

Teachers College, Columbia University
120th Street and Broadway
New York, N.Y.

Pediatric Rooming-In: Its Meaning for the Nurse

by CLAIRE M. FAGIN, Ph.D.*

There is a growing trend in pediatric discussion and practice for the mother to remain with her child during the child's hospitalization. This trend has profound relevance for nurses since it demands from many a change in both philosophy and role.

The purpose of this paper is to examine the topic of rooming-in from several standpoints: the rationale for rooming-in; the children for whom it is desirable; the mothers for whom it is appropriate; the role of the nurse; the role of the mother; practical considerations; and the current barriers against rooming-in.

As a background for this presentation, it should be pointed out that the author believes that rooming-in of mothers with young children is essential and that the findings of Bowlby, Robertson, and others, as well as her own, are more than sufficient to support this belief.

THE RATIONALE FOR ROOMING-IN

The consequences of a hospitalization experience for the emotional health of young children have long been of concern to parents as well as to professionals in the pediatric field. It is widely recognized that the continuous and contiguous relationship of the child to the mothering person is essential for healthy mental development in early childhood, and there is abundant evidence that separation of the young child from his mother can have negative effects on his emotional health. Bowlby,[1] Robertson[2,3] and others have described the emotional response to separation as well as the child's course in the hospital during the separation. Robertson has pointed out that the child of 2 "... appreciates

---

* Assistant Professor, Director of Graduate Programs in Psychiatric-Mental Health Nursing, School of Education, New York University, New York.

his mother as a particular person and has a hunger for her love and presence that is as great as his body's hunger for food."[2] He states further that "If, at the critical stage of early development when a young child has such a possessive and passionate need for his mother... he is admitted alone to a hospital... the child experiences a serious failure of that environment of love and security hitherto provided by his family which we know to be a necessary experience if he is to be a loving, trustful, and secure person in later life. He is too young to understand that there can be any reason... to justify the loss of his mother's care... For, at this age, the child does not reason—he feels and he needs, and the mother he needs so intensely... is not there..."[3]

A study by this writer[4] compared hospitalization of children from $1\frac{1}{2}$ through 3 years of age when the mother roomed in with her child and when she did not. Certain aspects of behavior were investigated before and after hospitalization. These were: reaction to temporary, brief separation from mother; emotional dependence; eating patterns; sleeping habits; toilet training and auto-erotic behavior. Comparisons were made of pre- and post-hospital behavior in each group and between the groups in order to test the following hypotheses:

1. Children who have been attended by the mother during hospitalization will not show a significant difference between prehospital behavior and post-hospital behavior.

2. Children who have not been attended by the mother during hospitalization will show a significant difference between prehospital behavior and post-hospital behavior in a regressive direction, and

3. There will not be a significant difference between the two groups of mothers in their attitudes toward child rearing.

It was found that children who were attended by the mother showed no significant regressive change between pre- and post-hospital behavior, and that significant changes in a progressive direction were found in several of the aspects of behavior cited. This indicated that growth was not impeded by hospitalization when the child was not separated from his mother. On the other hand, the children whose mothers did not attend them during the hospitalization showed marked regression in reaction to mother's leaving, emotional dependence, appetite, manner of eating, food finickiness, sleep behavior, and urination training. From the point of view of both child and parent, changes in hospital practice which permit mothers to room in seem clearly indicated.

It is interesting to note that in 1959 the British government published a report on this subject. This report, called the Platt Report, stated that parents of any hospitalized child should be granted *unrestricted visiting* privileges and should help as much as possible with the care of the child. It went on to recommend that mothers of children under 5 should be allowed, indeed encouraged, to room with their youngsters, and accommodations should be provided. Hospitals in Britain which have had more than ten years' experience with rooming-in of mothers have found that the mother's presence helps the hospitalized child recover more quickly and eliminates the problem of the distressed child at home afterward. This is pragmatic support of the previously cited study.

Child development theory stresses the child's need for his mother. There is wide recognition that until the child is about 3 years old his world revolves around his family, most particularly about his mother. She is the essential member of his family in the fulfillment of his needs and in the delineation of his universe. He sees her as omnipotent and able to control all events around him. He is absolutely dependent on her for much of his functioning, for protection and security. He is not able to understand what illness is and has no realization of time, so that the break, if the mother leaves him, seems final and irrevocable. It is known that many children feel that being sick is punishment for being bad. Being left in the hospital may be seen then as an even more severe punishment. In an experimental project with increased visiting and highly programed ward activities, it was found that younger children did not benefit to a satisfactory degree.[5]

Many studies have shown the traumatic effects of hospitalization on young children whose mothers do not stay with them during the experience. On the other hand, it is generally agreed, or at least there is no evidence to the contrary, that rooming-in of mothers with children in hospital allows the young child to handle the hospitalization experience with a minimum of trauma and that, following hospitalization, the child shows no adverse psychological effect.

FOR WHOM? FOR WHAT CHILDREN IS ROOMING-IN DESIRABLE?

The evidence points up very sharply that children under 5 comprise the group for whom rooming-in is absolutely essential. It is these children who are unable to benefit from preparation for the hospital, who are unable to understand time spans, whose need for and dependency on the mother is greatest, and in whom there is the greatest evidence of damage following hospitalization. The age of 5 cannot be a final limit, for many mothers of older children have reported problems following hospitalization. There is no systematized research on these problems, and further study is clearly indicated. Nurses and others should examine the effects of hospitalization on older children. For example, the adolescent who is having problems centered around maturation may feel his body image greatly threatened by a hospitalization experience. In addition to this threat, many of the emotions, desires, and fears of early childhood return to the surface during adolescence. Going to the hospital may evoke some of the same fears of separation that were discussed earlier in connection with the young child. It is axiomatic that the adolescent has the intellectual ability to deal with the realistic aspects of hospitalization but emotional problems may interfere with realistic appraisals. It is not possible to eliminate these age groups from concern without further study.

Some workers do not deem it necessary for infants to be attended by their mothers since the young baby with undeveloped visual discrimination will not "recognize" the difference. Therefore the baby may not suffer, if provided with warm and competent care. The necessity of further study is clearly indicated here.

It can, however, be stated unequivocally that most young children need the mother while in the hospital. Mothers of children under 5 should be encouraged to remain with their children during hospitalization in order to prevent traumatic effects from the experience.

SHOULD ALL MOTHERS OF YOUNG CHILDREN ROOM IN?

Many doctors and nurses seem to feel that they are in a position to judge which mothers should stay and which should not stay, often basing their opinions on the mother's apparent level of anxiety. There are many flaws in this practice. Perhaps the most basic flaw is that the mother, regardless of her level of anxiety or problems with her child, is the child's mother. This fact cannot be altered by the "superior" thinking of the medical staff. Actually, the child's need for the mother in a period of trauma may be inversely related to the quality of the relationship; that is, a child who is insecure and unsure of himself, and in doubt as to his mother's love, will feel even more rejected upon being separated from her when going to the hospital. This child will more likely feel that the situation is punitive than will the child who is secure and safe in the comfort and warmth of his mother's love. Robertson feels that mothers almost invariably do a fine job of concealing their anxiety when they are with their children. In addition, he feels that there is much more likelihood that the mother will appear anxious under restricted visiting, than when she can be with the child at all times and see and understand what is going on.

A point often made is that the child in the hospital is better off without his mother. The evidence cited for this is the frequency with which children's behavior changes for the worse during and at the end of visiting hours. At other times, these observers note, the child behaves quite well. It is important to recognize that the child's appearing "settled in" is not an indication that his distress is gone. Studies have shown that the meaning of the behavior is just the reverse of this. Robertson points out that the child often is in a state of despair which is characterized by increasing hopelessness. He is in deep mourning for his mother and his grief is of the greatest intensity.

Those who have studied this problem for the longest period of time believe that all mothers of young children, except perhaps those who are clearly psychotic, should be permitted, indeed encouraged, to remain with children during hospitalization. The professional person who believes this will assume some responsibility in educating parents to this point of view. In doing so she may find that some few mothers are reluctant to stay with their children.

What about those relucatant mothers?—the mothers who feel that they are not really important in the hospital; that they will be uncomfortable there; that it is not set up for them to stay; that people will say that they are keeping their children dependent. Should these mothers be forced to remain when their young children are hospitalized? After the nurse acquaints parents with the available evidence, which clearly indicates that mothers should remain with their young children during hospitalization, she will find that most mothers, when familiar with the facts, will choose to do the right thing for their children. The nurse's behavior must communicate to the mother a belief in these facts and a clear indication that the mother will be welcomed into the hospital society. Giving lip service to the idea but showing rather clearly by other forms of behavior that nurses would just as soon not have the mothers around will not encourage reluctant mothers to remain. Some mothers are reluctant to remain with their children because there are other children at home who also need their care. It is obvious that, in America today, if the mother can find no assistance in caring for these other children, and if the father cannot help in this matter, she really will be unable to remain with her child in the hospital. Pointing out to such a mother that she may come at any time of the day, evening, or night when she is able will do much to lessen her own anxiety as well as to meet more of the needs of the child than would be possible under traditional visiting hours.

In England, several mothers' groups working on this problem have organized baby-sitting services available to the mother who must leave other children when she visits her hospitalized youngster. In Edinburgh, the Mother's Care for Children in Hospital Chapter organizes and supports a children's playroom with a paid supervisor where mothers can leave their children while with the child in the hospital.

Despite all measures, there will be a few mothers whose reluctance is extreme and who will so resent an incursion of this kind in their lives that they are better off following their own inclinations. These will be rare.

What about the eager mother? Sometimes the eager mother may frighten the nurse even more than the reluctant mother; that is, a mother eager to plunge into the hospital activities may cause the nurse to feel, and sometimes correctly, that she will get in the way. Here the need for information is just as important as with the reluctant mother. The mother must have accurate information as to the child's need for her and the activities that are appropriate for her to carry out.

THE ROLE OF THE NURSE

The role of the nurse, in this context, can be viewed in three ways: (1) with the parents; (2) with the child whose mother is rooming-in; and (3) with the children whose mothers do not stay.

1. In terms of her role with the family, one of the important functions which the nurse will perform will be that of supporting the parents, so that they in turn will be able to prepare and support the child through the crisis of hospitalization. This may be done in several ways. Some hospitals have experimented with bringing the parents and the child into the hospital before the actual admission. This can be done most easily when a surgical procedure is planned in advance. In these situations, careful thought should be given to the content of the preparation. This will depend to some degree on the specific situation and the age of the child, but there are some generalizations that can be made. The mother and child should be oriented to the floor and room where they will be. The mother should be shown the physical setup of the ward itself: where things are, what the mother will be expected to do for herself, the kind of help she can expect from the staff and so on. She should be given some information about what will happen to the child when he comes into the hospital, as well as any pre-hospital procedures she needs to observe.

Enough information should be given to lessen the parents' and the child's anxiety upon admission, but not so much that they won't be able to absorb it. A little information concerning what to expect of the child postoperatively might be given at this time, but much of this can be saved until the child is hospitalized. The nurse will then review what came before and help the parent with the actual situation she faces.

For the unplanned or emergency admission the nurse's supportive role emerges even more clearly. It is best to have one nurse responsible for admitting the family and working with them on the unit. Her recognition of the mother's anxiety for her child and explanations of what she and others are doing and will be doing will help to remove some of the mysterious and awesome qualities of the hospital. The mother should help as much as possible with the initial procedures and in making the child comfortable. When this is assured, the nurse may consider with the mother a time for orienting her to the service. The essentials are the same as those described in the previous paragraphs.

The nurse's educative role encompasses being a role-model for the mother as well as direct teaching. When the mother feels the acceptance and understanding of the nursing staff she will be more likely to ask questions and seek help in areas of concern to her. The nurse is the mother's resource person. In addition, the nurse's observations of the mother-child interaction should be an valuable source of data for research and/or intervention in preventing physical and emotional illness.

2. The nurse's role with the child patient whose mother remains will vary in relation to the skill of the mother, the severity of the child's illness, and the complexity of the procedures involved. Her role as resource person will be constant but the specific activities may be different with each patient. Some children may not require technical nursing assistance, Here the nurse assigned will focus only on getting to know the family, observing the interaction, and meeting whatever needs emerge. Other children and families may require that the nurse perform only the most complex technical tasks and assist or supervise other tasks. There may be some children who require almost total care.

The nurse has to face her own "separation" problem from the child whose mother stays. Her role here is one step removed from the child. When she enters the room or cubicle she approaches a "unit"—that of the mother and child. Her recognition and acceptance of this unit affects her carrying out her role with the child and the child's acceptance of her. Her behavior must make clear to the child that she is there to help him and his mother and that she is not attempting to replace or displace the mother.

3. The nurse's role with the child whose mother does not stay is, for the most part, described in any good text or article on pediatric nursing. There are two differences in the hospital where rooming-in is practiced. First, the nurse will have the time to give the kind of care described since she will be assisted by mothers caring for their own children. Second, some questions may be raised by the unattended child as to where his mother is. With the older child these can be answered with relative ease. For the young child it is important for

the nurse to recall that these questions have always been asked by children. Perhaps it is easier for the person answering if a blanket response can be given to the effect that mothers are not permitted to stay. If so, to this degree the question becames more difficult to answer when rooming-in is the practice. Remembering that mothers who wish to room in are allowed to do so may also make the nurse feel critical toward the mother who does not, and she should be on guard against betraying these feelings to the child.

Recognizing one's feelings and seeking to understand the specific situation should enable the nurse to focus on the child and intervene in a helping way. The nurse's awareness of the anxiety-provoking nature of hospitalization helps in planning nursing care. For example, understanding the child's feelings of helplessness and isolation should determine the assignment of one nurse on a steady basis for each child. This nurse, responsible for the care of several children, will get to know their needs, know the information they have received and still need to receive, and be sensitive to cues of stressful situations.

The nurse's role with children whose mothers do not room in should in all cases be complementary to her role with the rooming-in families. Through both groups she is enabled to practice the art and science of nursing in its full scope.

THE ROLE OF THE MOTHER

It is evident that the mother's function is to attend her own child and do as much as she is able in this regard. Her purpose is to support her youngster through the hospitalization so that he can grow from the experience. Growth can occur under conditions of mild anxiety. With the mother present and the child sure of her continued support, anxiety is usually kept to a minimum, particularly if the mother receives the help described earlier.

The mother should be oriented to the idea that she is to help care for her child as much as possible—that this is why she is rooming in. She may make his bed, bathe him, take his temperature, help with his medication (if possible), and assist with many technical procedures. To the degree that the nursing staff accepts her presence and participation and helps her to help them and her child, she will. After a few days, if her own child is not critically ill, the mother may assist other children close by, performing a variety of useful activities. Here again there is a mutuality of roles. The nursing staff should acquaint the mother with the needs of the children and any rules regarding their care (i.e., fluids, food, bed rest, etc.).

The mother should be viewed as a full participant in the care of her child in the hospital. This is her role.

SOME PRACTICAL CONSIDERATIONS

There is considerable variation in the way hospitals handle the practical aspects of the mother remaining with her child. There is no real problem in providing accommodations for mothers, as most mothers would be willing to spend the night in a straight-backed chair for the privilege of being with their children during this time.

The actual sleeping and eating arrangements, fee schedules, and activities permitted and/or expected of the mother differ from hospital to hospital. Some hospitals provide cots for rooming-in mothers. These are compact and kept out of the way during the day. Other hospitals prefer easy chairs that convert into beds in the evening. In either case the mother may be expected to set up her own bed. Hospitals that do not have room or finances for beds for each mother may still permit the mothers to make themselves as comfortable as possible on whatever chairs are available. Although this latter approach is not ideal, most mothers will remain with their young children, despite the uncomfortable situation. In any case, the fee for the bed is usually nominal, starting as low as 50 cents a night.

Most hospitals that permit mothers to room in provide a food tray at reasonable cost. The mothers eat at the same time as the children and with them. Since the purpose of their remaining is to lessen the anxiety of young children unable to understand the meaning of hospitalization, their absence from the children should be minimal. In a large ward there can be considerable freedom of movement since the child is aware of the mother's presence without her hovering over him. In a private room where the child and mother are alone some thought must go into the mother's leaving. Even during the child's nap she should be nearby so that she may return when the child wakens. Some relief is generally provided during visiting hours when the father visits.

The mother's activities during her daytime hours might include (in addition to those previously mentioned) playing games and reading with her child and others; assisting with some ward routines; feeding her child and others; and any personal activities she enjoys such as reading, writing, or handwork.

Rooming-in can be handled by methods ranging from the most simple to the most complex and luxurious. That it need not wait for the latter conditions is being shown daily by several hospitals here and in Europe.

WHAT STOPS HOSPITALS FROM ALLOWING MOTHERS TO ROOM IN?

What are the barriers to rooming-in in pediatric hospitals? The idea has been discussed for years, yet relatively few hospitals have instituted the practice. Often reasons of space are given, yet many mothers would be willing to sit on a straight chair for a few nights.

Many observers recognize the similarities between the hospital and other kinds of closed institutions such as prisons. It sees its "inmates" as performing specific roles, geared to illness rather than to the needs of the total individual. Essentially, hospitals are economic devices rather than therapeutic devices, for it is obvious that in many ways the child would be better cared for if all the facilities of the hospital could be brought into his own home. The sharpness of the boundary separating the system from the rest of society stands in the way of change. This is not to recommend that there be no boundary but that some of the lines be blurred enough to allow the child to benefit from the ministration of both the family and the health facility.

Another problem lies in the delineation of or definition of power and responsibility within hospital structures. The power structure usually focuses around three groups: the medical group, the nursing group, and the adminstrative group. The medical doctors, although they are generally not employees of the hospital, are the individuals who hold the highest status. The nurses, though holding lower status, are employees of the hospital and frequently have some control over what goes on within the hospital. There is a strong tendency in this kind of system for professionals to "pass the buck" in terms of who takes responsibility for making changes. Physicians will often blame the nurses for not permitting progress, while the nurses await the doctors' "orders."

In actuality either group can initiate change if they feel strongly enough about an issue. If the other group resists the change, however, many problems ensue. For example, physicians insisting that mothers remain against the wishes of the nursing staff would invite not only difficulty in their own relationships with nurses but also an unwelcoming atmosphere for the mothers involved. This might doom the entire plan.

Another barrier to mothers rooming-in is the inherent change in the nursing role. The nurse is no longer the key person to each child but is one step removed from the child whose mother remains. In addition, her role with the family expands, and involves new learnings and competencies for the nurse. These alterations are bound to be met with some resistance, which needs to be recognized and met constructively by nursing administration.

A change of this magnitude, while essential, must be planned carefully. The planning should include all personnel who will be involved so that there will be understanding of the reasons for change.

The barriers to mothers rooming-in are continuously being removed. It behooves nurses to be initiators in furthering the removal of these barriers and in making rooming-in successful for the sake of their own growth as well as for the families involved. Nurses play the essential role in the success of the rooming-in practice during children's hospitalization. It is obvious that without their full participation the benefits of the program will not be realized. This partnership or triad of nurse-family-doctor augurs well for hospitals, for nursing and, most important, for the young child in the hospital.

SUMMARY

The need for mothers of young children to room in when their children are in the hospital has been discussed. Studies have shown that children under 5 regress in behavior when separated from their mothers during a hospitalization experience. It has been recommended that all mothers of children under 5 be encouraged to remain. The nurse's role with these mothers and children is primarily supportive and educational. The mother's function is to support her child and attend to as many of his needs as she is capable of.

Some of the barriers to permitting mothers to room in were described. These were the hospital as a "closed institution"; the power structure of the hospital; and the threat to "the nursing role." The new nursing role of initiating and participating in rooming-in projects was viewed as a positive trend for nursing as well as for the families involved.

REFERENCES

1. Bowlby, John: Maternal Care and Mental Health. Geneva World Health Organization, 1952.
2. Robertson, James: Young Children in Hospitals. New York, Basic Books, 1958, p. 8.
3. Idem, pp. 10-11.
4. Fagin, Claire M.: The Effects of Maternal Attendance during Hospitalization on the Post Hospital Behavior of Young Children: A Compative Survey. Philadelphia, F.A. Davis Co., 1966.
5. Prugh, Dane, et al.: A study of the emotional reactions of children and families to hospitalization and illness. Am. J. Orthopsychiatry, 23:70-106, 1953.

New York University School of Education
Washington Square
New York, N.Y. 10003

The Nurse's Reaction to the Ill Child

by BARBARA BRODIE, M.S.N.*

Nurses who work with children do it for a number of reasons, but primarily we work with children because we find them interesting, challenging, and satisfying. As one moves about in various pediatric settings it is apparent that many nurses are sensitive and perceptive to the feelings and problems of children and their parents when illness occurs, and they meet these problems with warmth and understanding. These same nurses display a fairly adequate background in the normal growth and development patterns of the child within the physical, social, and emotional framework. They do not usually find the noise, lack of routine and order, and hodge-podge of toys normally found in a pediatric area difficult or impossible to cope with. To be wet upon or burped on is considered all in a day's work. It is not always true, however, that these nurses possess the same sensitivity and perception about their own feelings. They may not even care to admit that they have strong feelings about any child or parent to anyone else.

THE FEELINGS WITHIN US

We are what we are for a variety of reasons—the sum of our experiences. We react as human beings to stimuli found all around us and regardless of how "professional" we think we are, many of the same qualities found in our young charges remain in us. That they do is not the question at hand; rather, the problem is recognizing them and learning to live with them.

Have you not met a situation in which a child deliberately did just the opposite of what you wanted him to do? Even after you (1) explained to him in terms he would understand; (2) spent time with him and his mother in establishing a rapport; (3) knew it was a neces-

---

* Assistant Professor, College of Nursing, University of Illinois, Chicago.

sary action for his well-being; and (4) could understand intellectually why he refused to do it and actually did the opposite, you find yourself doing a slow burn, becoming frustrated and peeved with the child and yourself. It's happened to all of us and yet how often have we explored these feelings ourselves or with others? Usually we mumble some appropriate comments such as "He's impossible, spoiled, too young to understand"—and then proceed to do it ourselves.

A case in point: Kenny is a large five year old who, although he had been in the hospital three weeks and confined to bed most of this time, suddenly began to soil his pants. He did it not only once but usually two or three times a day. He knew he should ask for a bedpan, for he certainly knew when he had to void. Yet regardless of what was said to him he soiled his pants. We knew he was expressing a need for attention, even negative attention, and so we spent more time with him but he continued to soil his pants.

Our most natural and quickest reaction as individuals was to feel angry and hostile with the child and in a measure with his parents because they didn't seem to be able to control the boy. There were many ways to express this hostility and anger. One of the younger nurses attempted to do everything for him and to give him everything he wanted except the one thing he most needed—to be warmly accepted for his own sake.

Others of us intellectualized about the problem, complained to the doctor or just sat around and bemoaned the whole situation. Never once did we sit down in a discussion period and analyze not only the group's feelings about the boy, but also our individual feelings. This does not mean that any of us were unaware of why the situation was occurring. But this was the way our feelings were being worked out.

Life has been described as "the licking of honey from a thorn," and certainly nursing is a profession which has its share of both honey and thorns. But what of emotions and their place in our lives? Most nurses will admit to emotions of a positive nature such as joy, happiness and the like. Few nurses will admit to negative emotions such as anger, frustration, or hate while dealing with their patients. But should we even judge emotions as being "positive" or "negative" in nature? Is not the very fact that we are human reason enough for accepting the presence of these emotions within each of us? Observation of a group of nurses gives little evidence that such acceptance is very widespread.

ANXIETY

Anxiety arises whenever we meet a situation which threatens our inner self or which threatens our concept of self and our relations with others. Although there may be actual external threats to us, the major portion of the anxiety is due to our inner response. For example, when a parent snaps at us about the fact that her child was to go to surgery two hours ago and we still haven't taken him there, we are beset by an inner conflict between opposing impulses and tendencies. We know that this mother is worried and upset, but she is taking it out on us when we have no way of controlling the surgical schedule. Our immediate response is to feel anger and anxiety but our intellectual and professional awareness of the reasons for this mother's behavior also makes us feel we must suppress these emotions.

Many times our perception of our anxiety is also blurred and varied. We may or may not "feel anxious," but one of the ways a person may feel anxiety is through feelings of anger. This anger may range from an overwhelming rage to feelings of irritation, exasperation, and annoyance. A nurse who cannot tolerate a mistake in herself may become very upset when an aide makes an error that is neither serious nor harmful.

Anger is so often the main component in anxiety that it is easy to understand why they are often linked in discussion. In many situations, when one becomes angry it is more appropriate to ask "What are you anxious about?" rather than "What are you angry about?"

Illness, hospitalization, loneliness, and the fear of the unknown provide more than enough grounds for our patients to become anxious and angry. The fact that we are often the brunt of this manifested anger and anxiety produces a comparable mixture of feelings within us. Our approach to these feelings, though, has been "professionalized." The nurse becomes quite cool, logical, and maybe somewhat condescending in her acceptance of these "outbursts" by the patient. This type of child or parent often is avoided, if not on a conscious basis, then certainly unconsciously.

Another way to avoid the personal implications of an emotional problem is to flee from it. The nurse who found the behavior of a 10-year-old so anxiety-producing that she called the building police to come to the floor and threaten the boy, stating that his delinquent behavior was simply beyond nursing, chose to avoid emotional involvement by making it a sociological problem and taking punitive action.

We can all match stories concerning the many forms in which anger can be expressed. But the point still remains that all of us experience anger and we will as long as we live. Anger is linked from an early age to an individual's efforts to protect himself from interference from outside forces. To reject the thought that you are subject to anger is to reject the complete understanding and acceptance of anger in a child.

HOSTILITY

Hostility is often an attitude that results from a situation that has produced anger and anxiety. The actual situation that created the anger has long since passed but hostility remains as a lingering or residual form of potential anger. This attitude may appear as a tendency to be sarcastic, prejudiced, defensive, suspicious or to strike out against someone (especially by way of a cutting and belittling remark) before he can strike you.

Again as individuals we seldom find it easy to admit that we possess and display hostilities. Many nurses learn to exhibit their hostility through a long list of grievances. Some complain about the doctors, administration, colleagues, and students. They gripe about salaries, the lack of help and supplies, having to rotate to different shifts, and the demands placed upon them by parents and children. Many of these complaints have a realistic note but one could speculate that the reason we don't easily find solutions for them is because we know they are legitimate ways to work off some hostilities. Hostility is certainly being manifested when a person looks upon everyone and everything else as being in the wrong.

Sometimes we may observe a child who acts as if we abuse him. In a sense every child in a hospital is abused to some degree. He is constantly meeting people in authority, being subjected to rules and routines that he would not impose upon himself and that often seem unfair and hurtful. All this comes on top of the fact that he is ill. Let us say he now becomes defensive and inclined to be smart and rebellious. This attitude is not calculated to bring out the best in the nurse and she may well become annoyed and angry. She may become short with him and otherwise punish him. Unfortunately a vicious cycle may be started that becomes very difficult to break.

Most adults have long ago learned that they cannot indulge themselves by expressing their hostility in the same way as the child often does. Rather, the nurse may use more subtle and disguised ways that are not as easily detected. She may become overtly solicitous and unwilling to do anything that may cause the child or parent to dislike her. At the same time she may be the very first one to pick up a little "gossip" concerning the child or his parents.

Identifying evidence of hostility, anger, and anxiety present among nurses should not be for the purpose of finding fault. What it should do is to encourage us to look at ourselves first as individuals and then as members of a profession. The longer we remain oblivious to the depth of these emotions within us the longer we face days of great frustration. Most nurses are intelligent, warm, friendly, and understanding people who strongly desire opportunity to help people, but too often the adjectives used to describe a nurse by the public are "cool, distant, aloof" and sometimes "abrupt and brusque."

LEARNING TO LIVE WITH ONE'S FEELINGS

When an individual is able to accept fully and freely the fact that she is angry and has a right to be angry she can begin to deal more effectively with the cause of her anger. Some of us, over the years, have actually given up the thought that we ever get angry. This does not mean that such people never get angry. In fact, they may be people who are extremely difficult to get along with. Their anger is either turned inward (as creating guilt feelings) or it may be handled by striking out against others. This we can see happening when a nurse will argue with a colleague who just happens to be a convenient target but had nothing to do with the original anger-producing incident.

Acceptance of oneself as a human being with a capacity and even a susceptibility for anger means that one can accept oneself even when one is stupidly angry, unjustifiably angry, cruelly angry, and foolishly angry. It is not an easy task to accept all of oneself, but it is necessary if we are to learn to deal with these emotions in a healthy way and learn to live with them constructively.

Nurses are quick to speak of the compassion component essential in the art of nursing, but compassion is inextricably linked to self-acceptance. To be a compassionate nurse one must be willing and able to accept the impact of any emotion. We must be able to enter into the tight emotional bond of fellowship with our patients when they are angry, fearful, frightened, or joyous. This bond requires us to feel and almost taste these emotions in their fullest meaning. I do not imply that the nurse should became equally frightened or fearful, for she hardly would be of any help to the child. Instead, she must know in an emotional sense what it means to be frightened and fearful. We must draw on both our experiences of and our capacity for being frightened and fearful.

A nurse who speaks about her understanding of why a child is frightened in the hospital, but does not go on to appreciate his feelings, really is not as compassionate as she might be. She must be equally willing to admit that she has known fear and will continue to know fear on occasion, in order to fully enter into his emotion. As she develops a sense of compassion for her own emotions she can truly be compassionate toward the child.

"But just what does all of this imply for me?" the nurse might ask. It has implication for both the student nurse and the graduate nurse interested in pediatric nursing. The student needs an educational experience that will help her develop understanding of herself and others. In the graduate nurse it implies that a process of self-examination should be instituted. The graduate nurse can make use of the opportunities for growth in self-understanding and human wisdom that she finds as she works with the children, their parents, and her co-workers.

Our conferences with our colleagues might well provide the opportunity to listen to and to speak of our personal problems as they relate to a situation involving a child or parent. We in pediatrics must develop some of the skills of communication our co-workers in psychiatry have found so useful. Many times I am struck by the fact that we seem to feel these skills belong only to the field of psychiatry where they are applied, therapeutically, to the mentally ill person.

The head nurse has a great deal to do with setting the stage for some constructive "give and take" among the staff. She should be encouraged to seek outside help, for example fellow nurses from psychiatry, a good social worker, or a psychologist who may be on the staff. Time should be provided in which patients and our interpersonal relations with them can be discussed in an atmosphere of ease and acceptance.

The subject of interpersonal relationships has come to connote the "winning friends and influencing people" concept, and often when speaking about getting along with people, it is assumed that this means pleasing everyone with whom we come in contact and being liked by one and all. This of course is impossible since we are constituted, by our physical heredity and environment, in such a way that no one possibly can entirely approve of us. In fact, there are many times when we ourselves do not entirely approve of us!

The problems involved in this task are numerous and difficult both for the individual and the group. I am acutely aware of that group of nurses who consistently work the evening and night shift. They often are the ones least likely to have any opportunity for a professional exchange as discussed above. The time the evening nurse has to talk with her fellow nurses is at best brief and limited many times to what has or has not been physically and medically done for the child. As soon as the report ends she is bombarded by questions from parents about their children, plus admissions and discharges.

The nurse who works these shifts many times is also a married woman with children who has really put in a full day's work before she ever arrives on the unit. All of these factors can, but *not necessarily do,* result in a rather harried nurse.

Staffing being a universal problem, we usually find this nurse is the only professional person on duty, although she may have auxiliary personnel such as aides or a licensed practical nurse. Therefore, she and she alone creates the millieu for the response of these people toward the child or parents. Often one has had the experience of overhearing a conversation among the auxiliary personnel that has been rather vehement about either a child or parent. Without too many questions or further investigation one will find that the graduate nurse has expressed comparable opinions and therefore actually set the precedent for this behavior.

THE EFFECTS OF EMOTIONS—POSITIVE AND NEGATIVE

It is not too difficult to see that how we feel about a child or his parent can have a direct effect on the quality of nursing care given. This fact has both positive and negative ramifications. I have primarily been discussing the negative aspects, but let us look at the positive side of the matter. Many children and parents stir up feelings of warmth, love, happiness, and contentment within us. Because of these very feelings we are more spontaneous in our giving of ourselves, and it certainly is no chore to be around these people. We easily accept the fact that we like these children and parents as people, and because of this we feel no inner conflict between our personal reactions and our professional reactions. Working in a happy situation that causes these emotions to be most prominent and acceptable actually encourages us to be very effective nurses.

SUMMARY

It can be said that nurses, because they are first of all human beings, must learn to admit that they experience many emotions and feelings toward people both on and off duty. Emotions are extremely powerful chemicals within the body, powerful enough, especially if denied or ignored, to actually affect our ability as an individual and a nurse. Nurses, like other people, do well in their profession because they have strong points, not because they lacks faults, and one such point is self-acceptance coupled with respect for self. A pediatric nurse who desires to be of help to the developing young child must be as honest and accepting of her own feelings and emotions as she attempts to be of the child's feelings. At best it is a difficult task but one in which the rewards are satisfying and encouraging.

REFERENCES

Bowers, W. F.: Interpersonal Relationships in the Hospital. Springfield, Ill, Charles C Thomas, 1960.
Jersild, A. T.: When Teachers Face Themselves. New York, Bureau of Publications, Teachers College, Columbia University, 1955.
Jersild, A. T.: In Search of Self. New York, Bureau of Publications, Teachers College, Columbia University, 1952.
McDonald, E. T.: Understand Those Feelings. Pittsburgh, Stanwix House, Inc., 1963.

4549 N. Kenton Avenue
Chicago, Illinois 60630

Administrative Responsibilities of the Pediatric Nurse

by IDA W. BALTIMORE, M.A.*

Administration is an important factor in the efficient operation of a hospital, and nursing administration is an integral factor in the activities of a head nurse. The administrative policies of a hospital are usually outlined in an administrative manual, which is standard equipment in each ward unit of the hospital. Knowledge of the policies defined therein can be very helpful to the graduate registered nurse who accepts a position in a pediatric unit.

"Pediatric" is a term that usually embraces the child up to and including 12 years. Exceptions may be those obviously well developed physically, and those in whom menses have begun prior to the 12th year. Some institutions have adolescent units to bridge the gap between 12 and 21 years.

There are divisions within the pediatric unit itself. These may include a communicable disease area, a tuberculosis unit, a section for premature babies (according to birth weight and/or period of gestation), a nursery for newborns in the obstetric suite, and an area for children who need long-term care. The last may include those awaiting placement when community facilities become available. Pediatric admitting and emergency units are usually separated from admitting and emergency services for adult patients.

All the above information is usually included in the orientation program for the new nurse when she is first employed in the hospital. She may have selected pediatrics because she "loves children," but the new nurse often has an inadequate concept of the essential administrative responsibilities that are interwoven with this love. Nursing administration is as much an integral part of nursing activities as psychological support is an integral part of the physical care of the ill patient.

---

* Assistant Superintendent of Nurses, New York City Department of Hospitals at Metropolitan Hospital, New York.

Yet many nursing schools preparing the student for practice as a graduate nurse omit courses in administrative or legal aspects of nursing. Although nurses who wish to specialize in administration usually continue their education on an advanced level, those nurses who wish to stay at the bedside, who do not wish to specialize, rarely have the opportunity to form an organized concept of the administrative responsibilities of the nurse. The bedside nurse must, therefore, look to her supervisor as a guide, and familiarize herself with the resources available within her unit which will serve as a valuable reference when the need arises. On the pediatric service some activities and equipment are merely scaled down to size, while others actually differ from those on adult services.

The following outline is designed to aid the nurse to develop an understanding of the basic administrative responsibilities involved specifically in the nursing care of children.

CONSENT

The child is usually brought to the hospital by a parent, other relative, guardian, policeman, or other adult. The admitting nurse is responsible for adhering to the administrative policies and procedures set by the individual hospital. The administrative manual is her guide. She must remember that parental *consent* is needed for admission and/or treatment of a minor. The signature must be that of the parent or legal guardian. It is obtained on an admission slip, and should be witnessed by the doctor. In an emergency, when time may be a deciding factor, exception can be made. This is arranged between physicians and hospital administrators, and does not come within province of the unit nurse. However, the nurse should be aware of the flexibility of certain policies, and use her judgment to notify her supervisor accordingly.

Knowledge of a foreign language peculiar to the locale of the hospital is often helpful in dealing with parents who do not speak or understand English. Interpreters should be utilized as necessary, and are usually available through the resources at the nurse's command. A fellow worker, another patient, or a visitor can serve as an effective interpreter, and often they acquire health information themselves as they assist the nurse by interpreting.

The parent must be properly informed of the circumstances and reasons for her signature. If the surname of the child differs from that of the parent, some pertinent notation on the admission record and chart can help prevent misunderstanding, loss of time, and frustration at a later date. Consent must be obtained for operative procedures and some specific treatments. Permission for blood transfusions may be difficult, if not impossible, to obtain if the parents are of certain religious convictions. Exchange transfusions for babies of Rh-negative mothers may be another instance in which consent is difficult to obtain.

Although the actual obtaining of the witnessed parental signature may *not* be the responsibility of the nurse, it *is* her responsibility to see that the consent has been properly obtained and recorded on the chart before the start of the procedure. This includes checking the date also. (It must be remembered that the chart is a legal document, and the nurse is responsible for maintaining accurate and detailed notes of all activities and procedures performed for the patient.) There are usually time limits for the validity of consent (example—5 days for major surgery and 21 days for minor surgery), according to the policy of the individual hospital. Should the time elapse, a new signature is required prior to surgery.

Occasionally it is necessary to shave all or part of a child's head in order to obtain access to a scalp vein for infusion therapy, or before a craniotomy. Consent must be obtained before cutting hair and fingernails in those cases in which family beliefs prohibit such actions before a specified age. Consent is also required for photography. This must not be overlooked, especially in burn cases which may later entail plastic repair. When a girl child enters the hospital wearing earrings which she may have worn through pierced ears since birth, it is wise to get written permission prior to removing them during hospitalization. The administrative manual should be consulted when in doubt concerning the need for obtaining consents.

Signatures are required for proper handling of property and clothing. The parent is encouraged to take both home, thus reducing the margin for loss or possible damage during hospitalization. Anything left in the hospital is at the owner's risk, and must be listed, signed for, and sent to the property office or clothes room. Upon discharge of the child, signature is again required for identification (by the same person who signed the child into the hospital) and for receipt of property and clothing. These signatures are essential as the first step in preventing later claims and time-consuming legal procedures.

EXAMINATION

The administrative responsibilities involving consent are important, but it must be kept in mind that the welfare of the child cannot be neglected while this "paper work" is completed. The nurse must examine the child carefully. His hair should be checked for pediculosis, and if present, it is treated promptly. The child's body should be checked for scars, bruises, extra or missing digits and any other abnormalities. If unexplained ecchymosis, burns, or possible fractures exist, the child may be a victim of the "battered child syndrome." The nurse must notify the social service department or the designated hospital agency, because this condition is reportable by law.

Sometimes a child has been abandoned or becomes ill in a public children's center and must be hospitalized. The nurse must be especially careful to observe and record details in such cases, since charts of these children may be requested for administrative review and often find their way to court. A detailed, legible nurse's note can be a valuable aid when the chart is reviewed in court, and often proves that specific nursing measures have been carried out. If activities are performed, or observations made, they should be accurately charted. An unrecorded observation is of no value and constitutes a basis for a charge of nursing neglect.

FEEDING

Administrative responsibilities may extend to the feeding of a child. When a child does not eat, it may be that he is unfamiliar with the food. It is not always easy to accept new or different foods, or even familiar foods differently prepared. The behavior and attitude of the child during mealtime may also be affected by his unfamiliar surroundings. Many hospitals allow "food passes" to be issued to parents if this will meet the specific need of the child and is not medically contraindicated. If a parent expresses a desire to bring in home-cooked food, the nurse should refer the parent to the proper administrative office where she may request this permission.

In many hospitals, visiting hours on the pediatric ward coincide with meal times. The presence of parents during the meal often shows a positive correlation with the food intake of the child. It also helps maintain some thread of family life during the hospital stay.

VISITING

While some institutions must hold to fairly rigid visiting hours, others have free visiting privileges. Still others have living-in arrangements for parents (see p. 83). This indicates that a real effort is being made to reduce the psychological trauma of a hospital experience to the child. The policy of the individual institution is usually found in the adminstrative manual.

When the parents leave after visiting, the strain of each parting can be emotionally taxing to both child and parent. Crying often arises by chain reaction. One child begins, the next one continues, and this can multiply until the nurse is silhouetted against a background of crying children. The nurse can do much to alleviate these episodes by providing psychological support to both parent and child during these critical periods. Although hospital administrators cannot turn off the tears, they can be advised if a specific policy or practice precipitates undesirable responses from parents or children. Administrative policies can be changed, and often it is the nurse who makes the observation and analysis, and then uses her judgment to maintain close interdepartmental communication. Her observation is often the basis for change and progress.

EDUCATION

When a child is hospitalized, his schooling may be interrupted. Most hospitals have some form of approved educational facilities for school-age children available within the institution. Sometimes a visiting teacher comes to the child's bedside. In some instances the Board of Education may house a bona fide public school within a designated area of the hospital. Children able to leave their beds or rooms attend classes there. Thus a child with a cast, in traction, in a wheel chair, or on a stretcher may attend classes. School instruction for the hospitalized child is usually planned on an individual basis. School hours and homework are designed to meet the needs of the individual child with consideration given to his handicap.

It is the responsibility of the nurse to plan medical and nursing activities so that the child will be ready to attend scheduled classes. The nurse should notify the school teacher if a new school-age child has been admitted, or if a child has special needs. The nursing care plan should also allow the child time to complete his assigned homework. The nurse should maintain interdepartmental communications and notify the teacher if a child cannot attend scheduled classes, or if his needs change.

RECREATION

Many institutions have playrooms for preschool children, as well as varied programs for older children. These include handcraft, painting, puppet shows, music, holiday and birthday parties, and special entertainment. Although the playroom is not under the direct supervision of the unit nurse, the nurse is responsible for working cooperatively with the playroom staff in planning activities for the hospitalized child. In the pediatric unit, bed rest is not synonymous with limited activity. Children with specific disease conditions may be allowed limited, modified, or full activity. The nurse, using professional judgment based upon knowledge of the pathophysiology of the disease process, should guide the playroom staff in selecting play activities for the hospitalized child. Many activities offer therapeutic as well as diversional value, and the nurse may help the playroom staff select toys best suited to the individual child. The nurse is responsible for seeing that the child is properly dressed and escorted safely to the playroom area by a member of the staff.

SAFETY

The nurse is responsible for the safety of all the children in the unit. Accident prevention and safety are of real concern to the pediatric nurse. The behavior of young children is often unpredictable, and children by nature are curious about their environment. An ambulatory child may explore his hospital environment and is thus exposed to many potential hazards. Bright-colored fluid in a glass flask, a hypodermic needle carelessly dropped on the floor, a sharp end of a metal bed frame, all invite obvious danger. More occult are the hazards of cross-contamination. One child may wander into the unit of another seriously ill child and become exposed to a life-threatening illness precipitated by exposure under circumstances in which his own body resistance may be at a low level.

The bedridden child is equally vulnerable to accidents. Climbing over the side rail and entangling himself in a jacket restraint are the more obvious hazards. However, when a nurse wheels a medication cart containing several medications into a unit and leaves the cart to administer a medication to one child, another child may reach out and consume or mix up the medications. A safety pin carelessly left on a bedside stand or a used syringe left within the reach of a young child may provide a potential hazard. These types of occult dangers are prevalent within any hospital unit and *utmost effort* must be put forth to prevent accidents.

Maintenance of a safe environment offers a unique challenge to the pediatric nurse. Campaigns are conducted periodically in many hospitals, with a reduced accident rate as the objective. Close interdepartmental communication and cooperation is essential in order to maintain an environment conducive to safety.

Good housekeeping is important. Clean, dry, uncluttered floors help prevent falls and broken bones. A conscientious porter who responds promptly when needed is a real asset. The nurse may request maintenance men to check window locks, keep window shades in good working order, and repair equipment. It is the nurses's responsibility to keep supplies in order in their designated places. Electrical connections should be protected and beyond reach of ambulatory children. Children sometimes trip over wires, pull out plugs, burn themselves on portable lamps, and even break bulbs and cut themselves. If there is a television set in the unit, it should be so placed that children will not be tempted to try to reach it to change channels

A child may easily lose his balance and fall from a footstool, chair or other equipment on which he may stand. Crib sides must be used judiciously for the purpose designed. If they are not properly adjusted, a child can easily fall to the floor and sustain a severe injury.

The nurse must always be diligent in stressing safety for the children. Although other personnel may supervise off ward activities, there are periods when children play in the unit. Use of materials supplied by the recreation staff may often require careful supervision for safety. Small objects such as beads, marbles, checkers, small pegs, crayons, clay, pieces of puzzles, or even a paint brush may find their way into a child's mouth or nose when the nurse has turned away momentarily.

Toys brought from home present special problems. Sometimes parents bring in toys with sharp edges, those that can be easily broken leaving a jagged edge or a rope or gun with which one child can easily injure himself or another child. It is the nurse's responsibility to guide the parents in the selection of toys for their child, based on his individual interests, activity limitations, and safety.

Children sometimes play in a rough manner or even fight. Such behavior patterns, although normal, may precipitate an accident in a hospital setting. The nurse is responsible for maintaining discipline in the unit, but discipline is not necessarily synonymous with punishment. Unit personnel cannot physically punish a child, nor should physical punishment be necessary. Often the correct attitude and approach by the nurse and ward or unit personnel can prevent behavior problems before they start.

The nurse must chart and report any unusually aggressive behavior of a child, as this may indicate the need for consultation, referral, or follow-up care.

If an accident does occur, it is necessary for the nurse to notify the doctor and her supervisor, and to fill out the required forms in detail. Accurate and detailed nurses' notes on the child's chart are essential, and preventive measures to avoid future accidents of a similar nature must be instituted immediately.

DISCHARGE

When a child is discharged from the hospital by the physician, the nurse is responsible for assuring continuity of care whenever necessary. Clinic referral, referral to a community agency, and interpretation of the doctor's follow-up orders to the parents are essential.

Prior to discharge, the nurse should return clothing and property to the child or parent and assemble the chart, which is later sent to the record room. Accurate and detailed charting concerning the condition of the child, and parent teaching regarding his care, is essential. Often the parent must sign a form and present identification before the child leaves the unit. The nurse should check with her supervisor or the administrative manual concerning the type of identification required.

SUMMARY

Nursing administration is as much an integral part of nursing activities as psychological support is an integral part of the physical care of the ill patient. Nursing administration in the pediatric unit presents many unique challenges for the practicing nurse. The nurse must use judgment based upon sound principles; she must utilize ward or unit personnel effectively; she must accept responsibility for all aspects of the care of the ill child; and she must know her channels of communication.

The nurse should familiarize herself with the administrative manual of her hospital and seek guidance from her supervisor whenever in doubt. A knowledge of the administrative policies of the hospital concerning admissions, consents, examinations, feedings, visiting, education, recreation and safety is essential.

REFERENCES

Erickson, F.: Reaction of children to a hospital experience. Nursing Outlook 6:501, 1958.
Leifer, G.: Principles and Techniques in Pediatric Nursing. Philadelphia, W. B. Saunders Co., 1965.
Marlow, D. R.: Textbook of Pediatric Nursing. Philadelphia, W. B. Saunders Co., 1965.
Miller, D.: Administration for the patient. Am. J. Nursing, 65:114, 1965.

Metropolitan Hospital
1901 First Avenue
New York, N.Y., 10029

A Physiological Approach to Pediatric Medications

by PAULINE F. TEPE, M.S., M.N.*

One of the most serious and important aspects of the nursing care of the ill child is the use of medications. The practicing nurse of today is aware of the demands made upon her by the tremendous advances in the field of pharmacology. Along with the benefits derived from these advances has come a greater responsibility for the nurse who has to administer these medications with intelligence and to observe and report the expected and unexpected results. This situation can become so complex and bewildering that the nurse often despairs of being able to function in this area safely and securely. When the patient is a child, the responsibilities increase because the child is different in his ability to communicate his needs and responses. In addition, the child may differ in dosage requirement and reaction to the drug because of some fundamental physiological variation within a particular age group.

A clue to at least a partial solving of this problem can be found in the basic fields of anatomy and physiology which form a foundation for the physical aspects of nursing care. In the area of pharmacology an understanding of these facts and principles is particularly important because drugs are designed to restore the normal physiological processes of the body which have been interrupted by illness. Logically, then, the nurse can develop a better understanding of pediatric medications and all they encompass if she analyzes them in terms of the anatomical and physiological processes of the specific age group for which she is caring. From this analysis follows a more complete appreciation of drug actions, dosages, routes of administration, anticipated results, and possible toxic effects.

The purpose here is to show by selected examples how a basic knowledge of anatomy and physiology can be directly and practically

---

*Graduate Teaching Assistant in Zoology, University of Arizona, Tucson.

applied to the nursing function of drug administration in the field of pediatrics. These examples will be drawn from three areas: (1) pediatric dosages, (2) toxicity of certain drugs, and (3) intramuscular injections. Although the intention is not to replace the standard safety practices inherent in the administration of medications to all patients, it is hoped that the reader will see how the area of drug therapy can be more meaningful to the nurse if she understands the underlying physiological factors. The development of professional nursing practice depends at least in part on such an approach, and can be accomplished only by the initiative and interest of the individual.

DOSAGES

Although the doctor orders the medication to be given, the dosage, and the route of administration, the nurse also shares in the responsibility when she measures and gives the drug. She should therefore have sufficient background knowledge to understand why specific orders are written and to question those she does not understand.

When only the adult dose is known, dosages for children can be calculated by various methods: according to age in months (Fried's rule) and in years (Young's rule), and according to weight in pounds (Clark's rule). Of the three, Clark's rule* is probably used most frequently. But most reference sources on drugs contain recommended dosages per unit of body weight for specific age groups and are frequently calculated on this basis.

In 1950, Crawford and others published a report stating that a more accurate and simplified method of calculating pediatric dosages is that based on surface area.[5] Some pediatricians are now using this newer method of determining dosage according to body surface area because they feel that surface area is more closely related than is weight to the metabolism of the individual. The smaller child has a greater surface area in relation to body weight and yet generates the same amount of heat per unit of body surface as does the larger individual. (It must be remembered that other factors such as growth rate and activity also influence metabolism at different ages.) Thus he has a higher metabolism per unit of body weight. And since metabolic rate is proportional to surface area rather than to weight, the smaller child has proportionately more active metabolic tissue.[2]

For example, the surface area of a 5 kg. (11 lb.) infant is approximately 0.29 square meter, while that of a 10 kg. (22 lb.) child is

---

* Clark's rule:

$$\frac{\text{Weight in pounds}}{150 \text{ pounds}} \times \text{Adult dose} = \text{Dose for child}$$

0.47 square meter, and the surface area of a 64 kg. (140 lb.) adult is 1.7 square meters. A comparison of these figures will show that the smaller child does indeed have more surface area per unit of body weight than the larger child or adult. If the nurse is interested in a further consideration of surface areas as compared to weight, she can find several nomograms that have been developed to show these relationships. The above figures were taken from a nomogram modified from data of E. Boyd by C. D. West.[9]

Table 1 shows an interesting comparison of dosages for selected drugs calculated both on weight and on surface area. In the table the surface area in square meters is expressed as M^2.

As can be seen from the examples, dosages calculated on the basis of weight and surface area are not always the same. It is also true that standard recommended or calculated dosages may need to be adjusted to the individual child's reaction. Prompt and intelligent reporting of unusual symptoms and the absence of desired results can aid the doctor in quickly altering the dosage to suit the patient.

There is controversy in the literature as to what method is the most accurate in determining pediatric doses. Other methods than the ones mentioned here have been proposed and as yet no definite agreement exists among authorities. In most reference sources that she might use, the nurse will find that dosages are listed for children of different ages as a certain amount of the drug per kilogram of body weight or per square meter of body surface. If she is unfamiliar with the dosage of a particular medication for a specific age group, she should calculate it on the basis of the child's weight before she gives it. She can also calculate it on the basis of the adult dosage using Clark's rule or one of the other formulas based on the child's age. If her answers do not agree with the ordered dosage, she has the right and obligation to question the physician. If he has used another method such as the one

Table 1

DRUG	WEIGHT and SURFACE AREA	DOSE/UNIT	DOSE FOR PATIENT
Kanamycin (systemic infections)	10 kg. 0.47 M^2	15 mg./kg./24 hrs. 0.5 Gm./M^2/24 hrs.	Total=150 mg. Total=235 mg.
Streptomycin (general use)	10 kg. 0.47 M^2	20-40mg./kg./24 hrs. 1.0 Gm./M^2/24 hrs.	Total=300 mg. Total=470 mg.
Digoxin (under 2 years)	10 kg. 0.47 M^2	Total Dig. Dose (O) .06–.08 mg./kg. 1.5 mg./M^2	Total=0.7 mg. Total=0.7 mg.

The figures for weight as related to surface area and those for recommended dosages are taken from Nelson's Textbook of Pediatrics, 1964. The total dosages are the calculations of the author.

based on surface area, she should understand why her calculations may differ from his. She must remember, however, that her answers will often be based on a total dosage for a 24 hour period and that the physician will prescribe the intervals into which it is to be divided.

DOSAGES FOR THE NEWBORN AND PREMATURE

Although average dosages for most children can be estimated by one of the previously discussed methods, it must be remembered that there are always exceptions, and one of these is the dosage requirement for newborn and premature babies. Usually doses recommended for infants under the age of 2 on the basis of weight or surface area are too large and can produce toxic results because these babies have not yet achieved physiological maturity. According to Kretchmer[7] the immaturity of the liver, enzyme systems, and kidney—all of which are involved in the metabolism, detoxification, and excretion of drugs—can cause prolonged action of the drug due to the inability of certain tissues to chemically inactivate the substance. Also the newly formed products can be toxic, or the active agent may cause an adverse effect in a metabolic area sensitive in the young infant.

One example of serious toxic effects that can be produced in the premature and newborn by a drug because of immaturity are those occasionally caused by chloramphenicol. The "gray syndrome" in these babies results from dosages that should be therapeutic based on weight or surface area. The findings indicate that the drug attains prolonged blood levels because of reduced renal excretion typical of this age group. Also involved is the immaturity of the liver and enzyme systems which detoxify and metabolize the drug in the older individual. Other drugs have been known to accumulate in the body to levels above those necessary for therapeutic effects for combinations of these same reasons. At the present time, probably less is known about the newborn's and premature's reaction to individual medications than any other group. The important general principle to remember is that they do not metabolize, detoxify, nor excrete most medications as well as children beyond the newborn period because of physiological immaturities. The nurse's awareness of these immaturities can be a protection for her patient when she is administering medications to this group.

Another interesting example of differences in dosage requirements is that involving digoxin. The recommended oral total digitalizing dose for a child beyond the newborn period up to the age of 2 years is 0.06–0.08 mg./kg., while that for a child over 2 is only 0.04–0.06 mg./kg. (It might be profitable here to remind the nurse that the total digitalizing dose is never given to any child at one time but is usually divided into three or four doses given at intervals of 6 to 8 hours.)

There is disagreement as to why the younger child requires more of the drug and several theories have been proposed. One theory is based on the previously mentioned principle involving surface area: Crawford feels that the younger child requires more digoxin because he has a larger surface area in proportion to body weight.[5] But here again the dosage recommended for the infant under 2 years of age is larger than that which can be tolerated by the newborn and premature. According to Robinson[8] the dosage for these babies should be one-half that recommended for the infant under 2 because of their extreme sensitivity to the drug.

TOXICITY

Since the area of dosages is closely related to the problem of toxicity, it may be beneficial here to discuss the correlation of toxic effects with physiological concepts. Paradoxically, a drug that is used to treat a particular illness or disease can also cause detrimental physiological changes as an undesirable side effect. These effects can either be related to the organ or system for which the drug is prescribed for its therapeutic action, or they can cause damage to another part of the body. For example, kanamycin is a broad-spectrum antibiotic which is effective against a great many infections caused by a variety of gram-positive and gram-negative organisms. But because it is excreted by glomerular filtration with no tubular reabsorption it can cause local irritation and damage to the renal tubules, especially in a poorly hydrated patient. This in turn can diminish the kidney's ability to maintain homeostasis of body fluids and electrolytes. Furthermore, in a patient whose glomerular filtration rate is reduced by other factors, the drug can reach high serum concentrations. Kanamycin also has a selective toxic effect on the auditory branch of the eighth cranial nerve and may cause irreversible deafness. The nurse who is aware of these possible detrimental effects should be alert to any subtle signs of deafness and any changes in the urinary output or appearance.

In comparison, the antibiotic penicillin is sometimes given to older children in dosages approaching adult levels. Although any drug can cause undesirable and little understood changes, penicillin has proved to be relatively nontoxic. The well known exception is the occurrence of allergic reactions ranging from mild annoyances to fatal anaphylaxis.

In regard to the previously discussed area of dosages, it might be mentioned here that the newborn and premature do not require large doses for therapeutic effects. This is apparently because the kidney does not function as efficiently as in the older child and this leaves a relatively high concentration of the drug in the body.

The previously mentioned drug digoxin can produce detrimental toxic changes in the heart. In a child too young to complain of nausea, dizziness, or blurred vision, the most reliable guide to toxicity is the appearance of arrhythmias.[8] The nurse should also be alert for a slowing of the heart rate much below that which is normal for a particular age group. If her observations and recordings indicate to the physician that a toxic level has been reached, he may want to discontinue the drug or lower the dosage. He may also wish to administer oral potassium if the toxicity is severe enough, since toxic levels of digoxin apparently liberate too much potassium from the myocardial cells following vagal stimulation,[1] and a certain level of potassium within the cells is necessary for adequate contraction of the fibers.

The three drugs used as examples of varying toxic effects illustrate an important principle in pharmacology: each drug is unique in its potential toxicity, and when toxic effects occur, they are manifested by detrimental physiological changes. The nurse who is interested in a sound knowledge of pharmacology will acquaint herself with all of the possible toxic reactions of each drug she gives. In regard to both dosages and observations of toxicity, the nurse assumes a grave responsibility when she interprets an order, measures the drug, and gives it to the child. But if she is aware of the basic physiological factors, she has a firm foundation upon which to build a fund of knowledge that will make her a safer practitioner. Only in this way can she begin to bring some pattern into the seemingly confusing matters of dosages for specific age groups and the occurrence of toxic reactions.

INTRAMUSCULAR INJECTIONS

The intramuscular route of administration is often used in giving medications to children of all ages because of its reliability in achieving accurate dosages and prompt absorption. The drug spreads rapidly along the connective tissue sheath of the fibers and is picked up quickly by the muscle's blood supply.

In the past, most intramuscular injections have been given into the upper outer quadrant of the buttocks, specifically into the gluteal muscles. Recently several studies have indicated the possibility of damage to the sciatic nerve when injections are given in this area to prematures, infants, and small or debilitated children. The sciatic nerve is actually a combination of two nerves enclosed in one sheath and divides into its two components in the distal one-third of the thigh.

As it emerges from the pelvis through the greater sciatic foramen it is covered chiefly by the gluteus maximus muscle. It supplies all of the muscles of the leg and foot and those of the posterior thigh, and contains sensory fibers from the skin of the foot and leg. Among the structures supplied by the lateral branch, or common peroneal nerve, are the dorsiflexors of the foot. It is generally believed that the lateral nerve is more frequently damaged than the medial tibial nerve; therefore foot drop is a common symptom of sciatic damage.[3]

In 1961 Gilles and French[6] published a report on an investigation they conducted on 21 cases of sciatic palsy in children ranging in age from newborn prematures to 11 years at the time of diagnosis. The cumulative symptoms were foot drop, gastrocnemius weakness, hamstring weakness, and sensory losses depending on which part of the sciatic nerve was involved. They claim that injections of certain neurotoxic medications, including many of the commonly used antibiotics, into or near the nerve can cause detrimental changes resulting in functional or sensory losses. This can occur even when the upper outer quadrant is used because of (1) the small area involved in the child, (2) the thin covering material provided by the gluteus maximus muscle, and (3) improper angling of the needle. To avoid damage to neurovascular structures they recommend that intramuscular injections be given to the infant, small child, and debilitated child into the lateral thigh at the junction of the distal third with the proximal two-thirds, utilizing the vastus externus (lateralis) muscle.

Combes and others[4] recommend the midanterior thigh as a relatively safe site for intramuscular injections for the infant and young child. Their recommendation was based on a study of 12 cases of sciatic damage presumably resulting from intragluteal injections. All of these 12 children were under the age of 2 and in most cases the damage was clinically demonstrated as foot drop.

A comparison of Figures 1 and 2 will show both the possible danger of intragluteal injections and the advantage of injections into the lateral or anterior thigh muscles. (The latter site is not one recommended by Gilles and French because of what they consider to be potential damage to neurovascular structures in the anteromedial area. However, a careful inspection of the diagram will show that no damage should result if the nurse is careful to avoid the areas through which the neurovascular structures run.) In many cases the specific area for intramuscular injections is either ordered by the doctor or is a policy of the pediatric unit or nursery. But if the nurse is thoroughly familiar with the anatomical structures involved, she will be better prepared to avoid injury to neurovascular structures regardless of the area which is used.

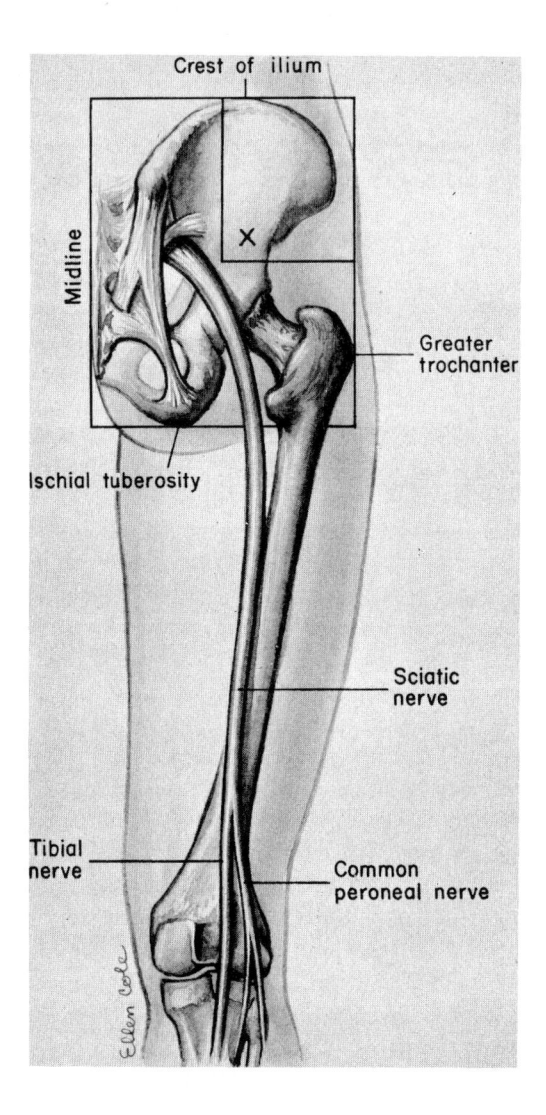

Figure 1. Diagram of the right sciatic nerve and its relationship to bony landmarks as it passes through the buttock. (From Chaffee, E. E., and Greisheimer, E. M.: Basic Physiology and Anatomy, J. B. Lippincott Co.)

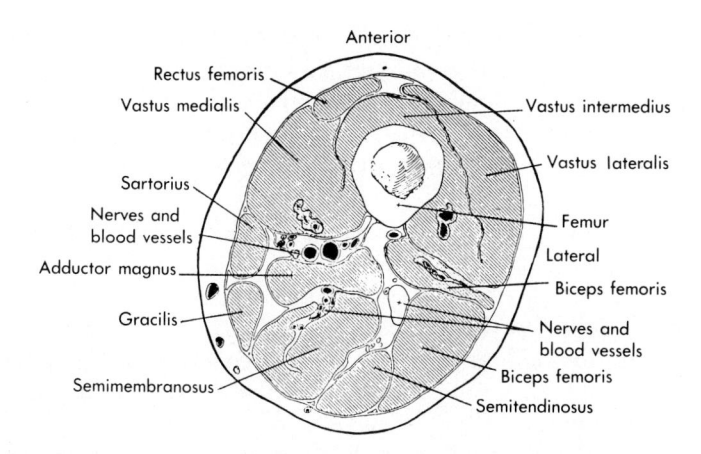

Figure 2. Cross section through the middle of the right thigh. (Modified from Eycleshymer and Jones: Hand-Atlas of Clinical Anatomy, Lea & Febiger.)

SUMMARY AND RECOMMENDATIONS

In retrospect it may seem that there has been an emphasis on the newborn infant and the child under 2 years of age. But this is natural because it is within these two groups that we find some of the widest variations in anatomical and physiological properties as compared to the older child or adult. The nurse must remember, however, that a child of any age can exhibit quicker or more toxic reactions to specific medications and she should always be alert to symptoms that may indicate this. Children have often been described as unpredictable and this is certainly true in regard to the area of medications. There is no rigid rule governing dosage requirements nor the individual child's reaction to any medication. The nurse who is involved in giving drugs to children should have an understanding of the following summarized points:

1. Drug therapy is designed to aid in the restoration of normal physiological processes which have been upset by illness or disease.

2. Difference in the anatomical and physiological processes of certain age groups will influence dosage requirements, routes of administration, and both expected and unexpected results of many medications.

3. Children of any age can respond differently and individually to any medication, often because of physiological variations that are still little understood.

4. There is at the present time a lack of knowledge concerning the

effects of many drugs, particularly the new ones, on the physiology of the premature and newborn infant.

Based on the above discussion and considerations, certain recommendations are now proposed for the pediatric nurse who wishes to establish a firm foundation upon which to build a better and more secure knowledge of drug therapy which can be utilized within her nursing role:

1. Have a knowledge of the basic physiological differences within the various age groups.

2. Analyze the anticipated results of a drug in terms of its effect on the physiological processes.

3. Be aware that a drug can have an adverse effect on the physiology or can cause damage to anatomical structures resulting in undesirable or harmful symptoms.

4. Keep a written record of each drug given, which can serve as a source of learning and review. Include the physiological and anatomical principles, therapeutic effects, usual route of administration, possible toxic effects, and dosage requirements for each age group.

5. Remember that, especially in the field of pediatric medications, a continuing study of pharmacology is both a practical and a professional necessity.

REFERENCES

1. Ainger, L. E.: Acquired Heart Disease in Infants and Children. *In* Brennemann's Practice of Pediatrics. Vol. III. Chap. 37, pp. 1-54. Hagerstown, W. F. Prior Co., Inc., 1964.
2. Best, C. H., and Taylor, N. B.: Physiological Basis of Medical Practice. 6th Ed. Baltimore, Williams and Wilkins Co., 1955.
3. Chaffee, E. E., and Greisheimer, E. M.: Basic Physiology and Anatomy. Philadelphia, J. B. Lippincott Co., 1964.
4. Combes, M. A., Clark, W. K., Gregory, C. F., and James, J. A.: Sciatic nerve injury in infants. J.A.M.A. 173:1336, 1960.
5. Crawford, J. D., Terry, M. E., and Rourke, M. G.: Simplification of drug dosage calculation by application of surface area principle. Pediatrics, 5:783, 1950.
6. Gilles, F. H., and French, J. H.: Postinjection sciatic nerve palsies in infants and children. J. Pediat., 58:195, 1961.
7. Kretchmer, N.: Practical therapeutic implications of immaturity. Pediatrics, 23:638, 1959.
8. Robinson, S.: Heart Failure. In Gellis and Kagan: Current Pediatric Therapy. Philadelphia, W. B. Saunders Co., 1964.
9. Shirkey, H. C., and Barba, W. P.: Drug Therapy. In Nelson: Textbook of Pediatrics. 8th Ed. Philadelphia, W. B. Saunders Co., 1964.

El Molino Mobile Park
1552 West Miracle Mile
Tucson, Arizona

The Nurse's Role in Fetal Medicine

by DORSEY IVEY SMITH, M.A.*

Man's universal concern for the welfare of the fetus has been displayed for centuries. Primitive art has been a mode for transmitting this concern, and researchers such as Margaret Mead have reported various cultural practices surrounding pregnancy and birth which center primarily on the well-being of the offspring.[4]

HAZARDS OF FETAL LIFE

In twentieth century life here in these United States, it still is not uncommon to hear such pronouncements as "the ingestion of strawberries during pregnancy will mark the developing babe" or "reaching over one's head will strangle the child." If credence is given to these statements, the pregnant woman may become truly frightened about her child. Regardless of the acceptance or rejection of these beliefs by the mother, no actual physiologic responses to such stimuli on the part of the fetus have been demonstrated. However, during recent years definitive research has shown the effects of various influences on fetal development, and the science of genetics has also made considerable progress. Three cataclysmic events have provoked the attention of a large number of people (lay and professional) and stimulated much of the research.

These events which catapulted fetal influences into prominence were: (1) the use of atomic weapons, which has evoked study concerning the effect of radiation on the fetus; (2) the Thalidomide drug tragedy, which produced so many defective and physically compromised infants; and (3) the rubella epidemic in the United States (1963–1964), which brought to light the impact of viruses on the development of human life.

In addition to these more dramatic fetal hazards, excessive smoking, an inadequate diet during pregnancy, and blood incompatibilities be-

---

* Instructor, Cornell University-New York Hospital School of Nursing, New York.

tween mother and child may also exert negative forces on the development of new life. Some authors are also postulating the effect of maternal emotions, especially as they reflect endocrine changes, on fetal development.[5]

The fetus is essentially a harmless parasite who derives his nutrients from his mother and also seeks protection from her. Besides the obvious anatomic structures which shield him, two devices peculiar to pregnancy are present. They are the placenta, which is thought to be somewhat selective in allowing substances to reach the fetus, and the amniotic sac and fluid, which will be discussed later.

Previously, the placenta had been thought to reject harmful elements, allowing only beneficial substances to reach the fetus. Presently to some extent this is still accepted in the concept of the "placental barrier." However, it is now known that:

"Transmission of materials across the placental barrier occurs by filtration, diffusion, osmosis, and 'pinocytosis' or engulfing. To pass across the placental barrier materials do not need to be of small molecular size. It is now known that molecules of very large size are capable of passing across the placenta."[5]

Consequently, more attention has been given recently to the effect of all the previously mentioned influences. With the exception of radiation, they possess the ability to cross the "placental barrier," producing deleterious effects on the fetus.

The role that heredity plays in leaving one fetus more susceptible than another has not been fully determined,[6] but one of the most obvious effects is exemplified by the predicament of blood incompatibilities between mother and fetus.

THE NURSE AND THE FETUS

Besides the evident need for continued research into human development and the causative agents in fetal malformation, where does professional responsibility, especially nursing reponsibility, to the unborn lie? Often, during his most vulnerable period of development, that of the first eight to twelve weeks of gestation, no one is aware of his existence. His mother usually is the first person who becomes aware of his presence, but often she may not acknowledge him until after these critical weeks, when he begins to change her physical appearance.

Since the mother provides the environment suitable for his growth, the nurse needs to make contact with her as early as possible. The public health nurse is often the first to do this, and hopefully she can assist the patient to locate medical facilities that will accept a woman carrying a very young fetus. Often this is difficult, since many women dislike seeking assistance unless they are positive about the pregnancy, and medical facilities tend to perpetuate this practice because many will not accept patients unless they have missed at least two "periods."

Frequently, therefore, teratogenic factors have already influenced fetal development before care begins. This is especially true of drugs, patent and/or prescription. Any medication is potentially a danger, and its lethal effects may have caused damage before anyone is aware of the fetus. The same thing may occur with the mother who contracts rubella early in the first trimester or who has certain bacterial infections such as syphilis.

Therefore the nurse, who recognizes that she may not be able to help the mother prevent damage during early fetal life, may have to concentrate her efforts on helping to prevent fetal damage before conception occurs. This can be accomplished by educating women to these latent dangers so that they can avoid teratogenic factors during the period when pregnancy is most likely. During menstruation and approximately 10 days afterward is considered the "safe period" when pregnancy is least likely. The remainder of the cycle is more vulnerable. Another appropriate effort in this direction is nutritional guidance so that the potential mother or host will be in an optimum state to nourish a fetus.

Secondary schools perhaps provide the best opportunity to reach the largest number of women within the childbearing years, and these educational responsibilities often fall in the province of the school nurse.

The nurse can also assist in formulating and implementing policies concerning the safety of pregnant women being x-rayed. Some principles to be considered are: the avoidance of x-rays (if possible) except during the "safe period"; use of a lead apron to shield the abdomen during x-ray examination or treatment; and postponing x-rays until the second trimester of pregnancy when possible.

The nurse should also remember to observe safety measures herself as she too is a potential mother.

MATERNAL-FETAL BLOOD INCOMPATIBILITIES

In the area of blood incompatibilities the nurse's responsibilities may differ slightly from the educational and preventive role that she assumed in protecting the fetus from the other hazards. The other influences that have been enumerated usually have their most pernicious effect early in fetal life; however, erythroblastosis fetalis may not affect the fetus until the second or third trimester of pregnancy. Hopefully, most women have sought medical care before damage occurs.

Incompatibility related to the Rh system is usually more deleterious to the baby than that affecting the ABO system.

The Rh system is now known to consist of several different antigens; the most common concept of the system divides it into three sets of allelic genes, C, D, and E, and c, d, and e. Various combinations of these genes can result in any of eight possible genetic types. Of all these antigens the D antigen is th most powerful; persons who have this antigen are those referred to as "Rh-positive," and those lacking it are "Rh-negative."

The incompatibility which most often causes erythroblastosis fetalis occurs when the fetus of an Rh-negative mother inherits the D antigen from his father. Because of the close proximity of the maternal and fetal circulations within the placenta, occasionally fetal cells with the D antigen cross over into the maternal blood stream. Anti-D antibodies are formed and these in turn cross back over the placental barrier into the fetal circulation and begin to destroy the fetal erythrocytes which contain the D antigen. The diminishing number of fetal erythrocytes leads to anemia and hypoxia and intra-uterine death may result.

The number of antibodies necessary to severely compromise the fetus may vary from individual to individual. However, previous immunization of the mother before the present pregnancy is usually necessary in order for fetal damage to occur. An incompatible blood transfusion in the past or another pregnancy may have served to immunize the patient. In the current pregnancy renewed contact with the D antigen may increase the numbers of anti-D antibodies and, hence, the chance of their crossing over to damage the fetus. The concentration of antibodies and their increase within the mother can be determined by taking dilution titers during pregnancy. In the past these values have served as a partial basis for deciding when it was medically advisable to intervene in the pregnancy. However, during the past ten years more definitive medical procedures have been developed.

The amniotic sac and fluid, as previously mentioned, provide protection to the fetus. Besides absorbing shocks and keeping the internal environment constant, the fluid can also be used as an indicator of fetal compromise in erythroblastosis fetalis. In this hemolytic disease the breakdown products of the hemoglobin, particularly bilirubin, are found in the amniotic fluid. Amniocentesis is one of two new procedures, and if this examination shows imminent fetal danger, the other procedure, an intra-uterine transfusion, may be performed. The fact that this hemolytic condition may be treated in utero serves to distinguish it from other fetal hazards.

The *amniocentesis* consists of direct aspiration of amniotic fluid from the cavity and spectrophotometric analysis of the fluid to determine its optical density. The optical density is increased if the breakdown products of hemoglobin are present. Based on this finding and the gestational age of the fetus, an intra-uterine transfusion may be deemed necessary. The fluid titers that are taken during pregnancy may serve to guide the physician in deciding the optimal time for doing the amniocentesis.

In the *fetal transfusion* Rh-negative packed red blood cells are injected into the fetal peritoneal cavity where the fetus absorbs and utilizes them to meet his vital need for oxygen. As a first step, the peritoneal cavity must be located by x-ray. Radiopaque dye is injected into the amniotic fluid and the fetus swallows this material, causing his gastrointestinal tract to be easily visible on x-ray and to serve as a landmark for locating the cavity. When this is clearly established, the physician passes a long pudendal needle into the fetus and a repeat x-ray is taken to determine the exact position of the needle. When it is placed correctly, the cells are transfused.

At present this treatment is reserved for the fetus who is expected to suffer intra-uterine death without it. If the x-rays reveal changes in the severity of the hydrops fetalis, then no treatment is instituted. For this treatment to have the most beneficial effect on the fetus it may need to be repeated several times before birth. These infants are usually delivered prior to term and normally require continued therapy after birth.

THE NURSE'S ROLE IN BLOOD INCOMPATIBILITIES

The issues raised concerning the nursing role in caring for patients with this complication are many. The author feels that the nurse may need to examine her own feelings and her beliefs about the manifestation of life in the fetus.

Patients often require information about blood incompatibilities and the nurse needs to be knowledgeable enough to explain them. Patients also may question the reasons for taking titers so often, or taking blood samples from the baby's father. These blood samples may help in predicting whether the fetus has a 50 or 100 per cent chance of inheriting the D antigen, based on whether the father is heterozygous or homozygous for the D antigen. Often the health of the fetus will depend on the mother's understanding of the need for continual care.

However, the more aware the nurse is of her own feelings, the easier it may be for her to cope with helping the patient to reach her own answer to the following questions: "Nurse, what should I decide? I just don't know whether to let them do anything to the baby or not"; or "Do you really think all this treatment will be worth it to the baby?" Patients may ask these questions even after the physician has carefully explained the risks. Deciding on intra-uterine transfusion is not easy, as many risks are involved and no guarantee can be given as to the fetal outcome. Because the nurse is considered a "significant person" by patients and because her attitudes are conveyed by both verbal and nonverbal modes of communication, she is in essence a "significant person" to the unborn being.

AMNIOCENTESIS

If amniocentesis is required, the patient needs to understand the reason for remaining still during the procedure. It is essential that she do so, to prevent the needle from becoming misplaced. The physician doing the procedure first palpates the mother's abdomen to locate the position of the fetus and then introduces a long pudendal needle into a space within the amniotic cavity best located for avoiding both the fetus and placenta. The amniotic fluid is then aspirated and the needle removed.

This may or may not be done under local anesthesia; however, in both cases patients have stated that they feel more pressure than pain, but that anticipation of the event makes it difficult to remain still. Nursing measures which may help a patient to remain still are: staying beside the patient's head, holding her hands, verbal encouragement, and mopping her brow if necessary.

After the aspiration, checking the fetal heart rate and taking the patient's blood pressure are important factors. If fetal distress is noted and the infant is large enough for possible survival, immediate delivery may be considered. Occasionally, a patient may have a significant decrease in blood pressure. If this is due to hemorrhage from the placenta, again more extreme medical measures may need to be taken. Amniocentesis is frequently done on an outpatient basis so that these observations must be made fairly rapidly following it. Instructing the patient to contact the hospital if she perceives changes in fetal activity is important.

INTRA-UTERINE TRANSFUSION

When a patient is admitted for an intra-uterine fetal transfusion, analgesic and hypnotic drugs may be ordered "on call" for the patient. These drugs are administered to assist in relieving some of the anxiety patients usually experience, and to help them in the task of remaining still during the procedure. The latter factor is especially important here as the needle must remain in the fetal peritoneal cavity. Prior to the procedure, food and fluid by mouth may be withheld for several hours to prevent the possibility of aspiration.

During the transfusion, the nurse again can assist the patient by remaining with her, by physical contact, and by continuously giving her step by step information. Because of the sedation a patient will sometimes drift off to sleep, but may awaken abruptly. This may cause her to move. If a nurse is alert to this possibility, she can caution the patient not to move. Measures such as a cool cloth to the head and wet compresses to the lips can relieve some discomforts of the procedure.

After the transfusion the fetal heart may be checked, but again the physicians will consider many factors before intervening for fetal distress. However, untoward maternal blood pressure readings may be more significant in requiring medical attention. At this time, too, an antibiotic drug is often ordered as a prophylactic measure against infection, and nursing observations, especially of the temperature and pulse, become exceedingly important. A back rub is often very refreshing for patients, as lying on one's back for extended periods is difficult.

DELIVERY IN CASES OF MATERNAL-FETAL INCOMPATIBILITY

When an iso-immunized patient is admitted for delivery, the nurse needs to be aware of this fact in order to make special arrangements for the fetus. This is especially necessary in preparing for the birth of a transfused infant. Usually these infants are delivered several weeks prior to term and are expected to be ill at birth as well as premature. Resuscitation at birth should be anticipated.

The two main areas for these special arrangements are in preparing equipment for resuscitation, for safe transportation of the infant, and for collecting additional cord blood specimens, and in communicating with other members of the health team, particularly the pediatrician and the nurse in the premature nursery, so that they too can prepare to care for the child.

The blood tests which are done on the infant include a Coombs test, measurement of nucleated red blood cells, a hematocrit determination and, soon after birth, a bilirubin determination. These all are indicative of the baby's hematologic status and are guides to further therapy.

The nursing observations made both at birth and regularly in the premature nursery include respirations, color, activity, and muscle tone. The condition of the cord and the skin of the abdominal wall is checked. Hematomas from the transfusions are prevalent, and prevention of hemorrhage is extremely important in these infants. The usual handicaps displayed by premature infants are evident, and at birth these babies appear especially pale and anemic. These observations are helpful in assessing the infant's adjustment to life and to his disease.

Because mother and baby are separated physically and because the health status of the infant may be questionable, the nurse needs to promote a healthy mother-child relationship by providing the opportunity for the mother to visit and to ask questions about the condition

Name				Birth Date			History Number			
Lab. Tests										Dates
Coombs				Mother's Bl. Type			Fetal Transfusions:			
Bilirubin				Hx. No.			Exchange Transfusions:			
Blood type							"Booster" Transfusions:			
Date	Wgt.	Temp.	Cord	Skin	Urine	Stool	Color	Muscle Tone	Activity	Resp.

	Temp.	Humidity	Oxygen
Isolette			
Incubator			
Crib			

Feeding	Check	Date	Intake
NPO			
Intravenous			
Gavage			
Formula			

Mother-Child Relationship	Nursing Intervention Measures

Figure 1. Example of a nursing care plan that can be utilized in caring for babies that have had fetal transfusions. Only the main points are enumerated, but for a useful record additional space would be required for many of the items.

of her child. The nurse can also assist the mother in having physical contact with her baby as soon as this is possible.

Exchange and/or "booster" transfusions may be needed during early life. After discharge, medical follow-up is of the essence, so that additional transfusions may be given on an outpatient basis, as needed. The nurse can play a significant role here in explaining the necessity for keeping these appointments and may also encourage the mother to keep her own post-partum check-up appointment.

CONCLUSIONS

Fetal medicine is just coming into being, and nursing is beginning to shape its role in promoting the well-being of early human life. The knowledge that a nurse requires in order to fulfill this responsibility comes from many disciplines. In the basic sciences a knowledge of genetics, embryology, and physiology is needed. In nursing, knowledge of both pediatric and maternity nursing is essential, for one cannot say arbitrarily that the fetus belongs exclusively to either segment. These two aspects of nursing, which are so close, yet often find themselves so far apart, thus have another link. The broad areas of nursing responsibility within this emerging specialty are education, observation, support, and anticipatory guidance. The nurse can do much to promote the welfare of both mother and fetus, and to preserve the precious gift of a new human life.

REFERENCES

1. Apgar, Virginia: Drugs in pregnancy. Am. J. Nursing, 65:104–105, 1965.
2. Freda, Vincent, and Robertson, John: Amniotic fluid analysis in Rh isoimmunization. Am. J. Nursing, 65:64–68, 1965.
3. Glynn, Elizabeth: Nursing support during intra-uterine transfusion. Am. J. Nursing, 65:72–73, 1965.
4. Mead, Margaret: Male and Female. New York, William Morrow & Co., 1949.
5. Montague, Ashley: Prenatal Influences. Springfield, Ill., Charles C Thomas, 1962.
6. Nishimura, Hideo: Chemistry and Prevention of Congenital Anomalies. Springfield, Ill., Charles C Thomas, 1964, Chapter II.
7. Queenan, John: Intra-uterine transfusion for erythroblastosis fetalis. Am. J. Nursing, 65:68–71, 1965.
8. Queenan, John, and Adams, Daniel: Multiple intrauterine transfusions for erythroblastosis fetalis. Obst. & Gynec., 25:302–307, 1965.
9. Queenan, John, and Gordon, Douglas: Amniocentesis for prenatal diagnosis of erythroblastosis fetalis. Obst. & Gynec., 25:308–321, 1965.

1 Garrett Place
Bronxville, New York

Hyperbaric Oxygenation: Nursing Responsibility in Planning for a New Clinical Service

by MARY JANE VENGER, M.A.*

The Director of Nursing must assume a leadership role in the planning for a new clinical facility with the administration and the physician. An ideal opportunity to demonstrate this principle occurred when I was invited to the preplanning conferences of the Medical Committee on Hyperbaric Oxygenation. This challenge was a real one because it was concerned with a relatively new avenue for nursing care of patients as well as the experimental endeavors in a hyperbaric chamber.

Hyperbaric oxygenation can be defined as the administration of oxygen in an environment of increased atmospheric pressure. This procedure permits more oxygen to be dissolved in the body fluids, in the same way that more gas becomes dissolved in a soft drink bottled under pressure. When a person breathes 100 per cent oxygen in a chamber in which the atmospheric pressure is three times normal, approximately 20 times as much oxygen as normal is dissolved in the blood plasma. This form of therapy has been effective in producing lifesaving cures in gas gangrene, tetanus, and carbon monoxide poisoning. Its potential in surgery for patients who ordinarily could not withstand operation is limitless. Its use in cardiac and other cardiovascular conditions remains to be explored.

HISTORY

Historically, pressure chambers are not new. It is reported that the concept of increased atmosphere as a therapeutic milieu goes back

---

* Director of Nursing, Mount Sinai Hospital, New York.

to the days of Aristotle. The Problemata of Alexander (332 B.C.) mentions a diving bell. Robert Boyle, the English physicist, in 1659 was the first to show that a "vital material" in the air (oxygen) was ncessary for maintaining life. His experiments demonstrated bubbles of gases which appeared in the tissues of animals if they died under conditions of decreased (hypobaric) ambient pressure. The discovery of oxygen by Priestley occurred in 1775. It is reported that the first caisson for underwater construction work was developed by Triger, a Frenchman, in 1841. This was a "first" in the application of hyperbaric conditions. A surgical procedure was reported to have been done under mild degrees of hyperpressure by Dr. Pravaz, a Hungarian surgeon, in 1843. In modern times, the pioneer contributions of Wangensteen and Lovelace in 1941 included the application of hyperpressure in a pressure vessel for bowel obstruction.

FIRST STEPS IN PLANNING

The initial step in planning was to define, identify, and learn the principles of a hyperbaric atmosphere, the use of oxygen and the chamber. It was necessary to disseminate information about the proposed project to the entire nursing staff so that genuine interest would result when recruits were sought for the group planning nursing care for the potential patients. The available literature was disseminated and a general information discussion was planned for each level of the professional nursing staff. Visits were made by nurses to the existing installations at the Western Infirmary, Glasgow, Scotland, the Wilhelmina Gasthus in Amsterdam, The Netherlands, and the Lutheran General Hospital in Chicago. During these visits discussions were held with the medical and nursing staffs regarding their experiences in developing and implementing their respective programs. It became apparent that nursing must have a definitive role in planning with the physician, ancillary services, and administration. Leadership by nursing in this instance was to be the challenge; the answer was to be establishment of an organized nursing unit.

As a result of the literature and discussions made available to the staff, a group of professional nurses volunteered to become members of an advisory committee which began the planning and organization of the nursing unit. This group visited the Linde Oxygen Division of Union Carbide at the time when the chamber was being built. It was an important step for the staff to be able actually to inspect the structure. There were discussions with the engineers and technicians who were involved in developing the intricacies of the vessel.

At the same period, many nurses attended a three-day institute on hyperbaric oxygenation organized by the New York and National Academies of Sciences in conjunction with members of our medical staff. This provided opportunity for our nurses to gain greater insight and understanding of the experiences with as well as the processes and problems of hyperbaric oxygenation.

WORK OF THE NURSING ADVISORY COMMITTEE

The process of identifying the needs of potential patients pointed up the necessity to involve many other representatives of the hospital family who contribute to the total patient care. To meet basic needs and provide services such as linen, drugs, housekeeping, transportation, engineering, inhalation therapy, anesthesiology, medical records, etc., invitations were extended through administration and the Medical Committee on Hyperbaric Oxygenation.

The nursing needs were divided into two major areas: (1) selection and staffing, (2) staff development. It was decided that for nurses who were interested and who might become involved a basic staff development program should be initiated. First it was necessary to identify a basic nursing philosophy, and policies and procedures that would be appropriate and meaningful to this expanding horizon of nursing practice. We decided that the nursing role would be complex, with great responsibility placed on the knowledge, skill, and judgment of the nurse. For example, lifesaving measures usually initiated and carried out by physicians were taught to us (Fig. 1). These procedures would have to be done by nurses in the chamber when the physician is on rounds, in the control area, or in his office. Because of the time needed for decompression and compression, no one else can enter the chamber to handle emergencies, but closed television and intercom systems makes it possible to see and talk with the physician.

A symposium on basic physics was conducted by Dr. Trygve Jensen, professor of chemistry and physics and author of a physics textbook for nurses.[1] This program was essential to group understanding of our own basic procedures and policies.

Chamber operations were discussed by the technicians who operate the hyperbaric unit. These men have had extensive diving experiences, and are competent in the use of the Navy decompression tables.[2] Their understanding of the application of fire-fighting apparatus, the other types of hazards and general protocol to be observed when the chamber is under pressure, as well as potential complications (such as the "bends"), was invaluable.

After some months of experience, the nursing staff of the unit presented a program to the entire nursing personnel on their experiences in the chamber.

THE MOUNT SINAI HOSPITAL
HYPERBARIC OXYGENATION UNIT

EMERGENCY PROCEDURE EXPERIENCE RECORD FOR NURSES

NAME: _____

PROCEDURE	INSTRUCTION BY	DATE	PRACTICE SUPERVISED BY (SIGNATURE)	DATE
Application of Defibrillator				
Application of External Pacemaker				
Use of Ambu Resuscitator				
Use of Bird Respirator				
Venipuncture				
Insertion of Nasogastric Tube				
Reduction of Pneumothorax by Needle Insertion				
External Cardiac Massage				
Deep Tracheal Suction				
Introduction of Oral Airways				
Introduction of Endotracheal Tube				
Collection of Blood Specimens via Arteriotomy				
Lab. Tests: Arterial pO_2, pCO_2, pH (Astrip)				
Use of Pressor Infusor for Transfusions				
Initiation of Infusions of Blood Plasma Albuminosol				
Application of Hypo-hyperthermia Apparatus				
Inflation of Cuffed Tracheostomy Tubes				

Figure 1. Form showing procedures taught to nurses who will work in the hyperbaric oxygen chamber.

THE NURSING STAFF AND NURSING CARE

The Hyperbaric unit at Mount Sinai Hospital is a multipurpose unit designed to function as an experimental laboratory, an operating room (Fig. 2), and a medical treatment facility. These purposes defined

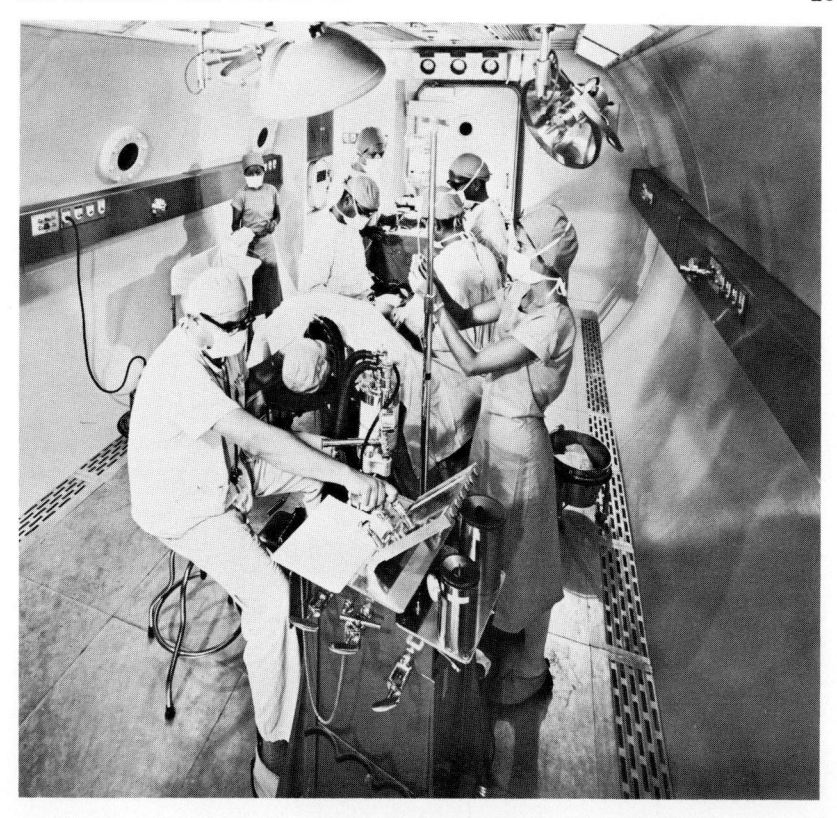

Figure 2. An operating room team at work in the hyperbaric oxygen chamber at Mount Sinai Hospital.

for us the kinds of talents that would be needed in the nursing staff. It was determined that experience in operating room nursing and intensive care should serve as qualifications of the candidate. Selection was made on the basis of proficiency of nursing practice, general attitude, interest, and endurance, as well as the potential ability to attempt to meet changing needs and emergencies. All personnel were subjected to a rigorous physical examination conducted by the Employees Health Service. Figure 3 shows the check list employed for medical evaluation.

As the nursing staff began their planning sessions with representatives of administration, clinicians, and ancillary services, the quality of patient care became identified as individual to the program. Principles were developed as guidelines. We had the opportunity to "practice" in a real situation where critically ill patients "as a last resort" were administered hyperbaric oxygenation in the experimental chamber. These "dry runs" offered the nursing staff, administration, and ancillary services the opportunity to develop from our discussion immediate plans to

MEDICAL EVALUATION CHECK LIST FOR HYPERBARIC PERSONNEL

Name	Age	Weight	Height	Unit #

TEST:	Date Scheduled	Date Completed	Dates of Follow-up Work
1. Physical Examination			
2. ENT Examination			
3. Audiogram			
4. Sinus X-rays			
5. Chest X-ray			
6. Hematocrit			
7. WBC			
8. Urinalysis			
9. ECG			
10. EEG			
11. Visual Fields			
12. Visual Acuity			
13. Dental X-rays			
14. Long Bone X-rays			

N = Normal
U = Unchanged
A = Abnormal but not disqualifying
D = Disqualifying if uncorrected or correctable

Grant Number _____
Bill to: _____
Date Billed _____
Payment Received _____

Figure 3.

HYPERBARIC OXYGENATION

THE MOUNT SINAI HOSPITAL
NEW YORK
HYPERBARIC OXYGENATION
CONSENT FOR PROCEDURE

| DATE |
| LOCATION |
| NAME |
| UNIT NO. & SEX AGE |
| PHYSICIAN & SERVICE |

Hyperbaric oxygenation therapy has been explained to me. I fully understand that it may involve some unknown and unforeseen risks. With this knowledge and the explanation given, I voluntarily accept the risk and realize that this procedure will not necessarily result in cure or improvement. In view of the mutual understanding and purpose, I therefore agree to hold Dr. _____ _____, and his associates, and the Mount Sinai Hospital and those associated therewith free of liability for results of the procedure.

_____   _____
Witnessed By   Patient's Signature

_____   _____
Title   Date

I, the undersigned, have defined and fully explained the studies involved to the above patient.

_____
Investigator's Signature

_____
Date

10/8/64

Figure 4. Form for consent to procedure.

organize, coordinate and then to evaluate the effectiveness of setting up a nursing area and administering care under "atypical conditions." The policies and procedures that evolved out of these experiences have been invaluable to the staff.

First and foremost, the nurse must be an observer attuned to the inherent individuality of hyperbaric oxygenation; i.e. she must recognize early signs of oxygen toxicity, air embolus, spontaneous pneumothorax, or simply claustrophobia.

Emotional support of a patient and his family is a prime responsibility of a nurse in any setting. Since this whole concept of therapy is new to everyone, including many medical personnel, it is imperative that nurse and physician collaborate in offering an explanation to the family and patient. Inasmuch as a consent (Fig. 4) for this therapy is necessary,

INTERPRETATIONS OF PATIENT REACTIONS

For each item listed please indicate if there was any deviation from the usual or expected response and if so describe briefly.

Note whether response was verbalized by patient or observed by nurse.

		Response
I	Temperature	100.4
	Pulse	92 Taken by Miss Smith
	Respiration	24
II	Pain	Continues to be present in chest area
	Nausea	None
	Congestion	To be checked by physician
	Dizziness	None noted
	Numbness	None noted
	Muscular weakness	Patient complains of this in lower extremities
	Incoordination	Not noted
	Extremities-(tingling) (floating)	Not noted or reported
	Irritability	Not noted
	Restlessness	Appears so at frequent intervals
	Lip twitching	Noticeable
	Batting of eyelids	Infrequently noted
	Tremor	Observed once in past 4 hours – 8 p.m.
	Choking sensation	Not noted
	Itching-(burning) (rash)	Not reported
III	Vision	⎫
	Hearing	⎪
	Voice	⎬ No change
	Touch	⎪
	Smell	⎭
	Taste	
	Hunger	
	Thirst	Apparently increasing
IV	Fatigue	Continuously expressed by the patient
	Depression	Appears to some degree
	Level of alertness	Poor
	Fear	⎫ Appears to be both
	Anxiety	⎭
	Feeling of well being	⎫ No change of note
	Euphoria	⎭
	Concentration	Depressed to some extent
	Mood	
	Reaction to others	⎫ Evidenced by wakefulness
	Awareness of individuals outside of chamber	⎭
	Need to talk	⎫ Not applicable
	Need for recreation	⎬
	Sudden apprehension	⎭

Figure 5. Example of log of patient reactions during hyperbaric oxygen treatment.

Figure 5. *continued*
- 2 -

V   Interest in procedure
      Number of exposures
      Hour of exposure
      Number of exposures during past 12 hours   *150 minutes*
      Passage of time
      Effect of noise

VI   Diaphoresis
      Elimination
        Bladder
        Bowel   *No change*
      Secretions
        Nasal
        Salivary
        Tracheal

Factors which may have influenced reactions:
    Age of patient   *42*
    Diagnosis
    Physical condition   *Not determined*
    Sedation

Comments:

Modifications of Nursing Care due to Hyperbaric Oxygenation

Ability to care for patient in usual manner
    Activity and effort required
Any difference in needs of patient while in the Hyperbaric chamber
    Amount of time spent providing physical care
    Amount of time spent providing emotional support
      Active
      Passive
Change of approach to meet patient needs
Groups in therapy
    Communications between patients
    Differences of response of patients when more than one in therapy

---

the time of obtaining this provides an excellent opportunity to give added support. The fact that nurse, doctor, and patient are exposed to the same environment and share many of the same stresses and strains seems to give the patient an increased sense of security. This sharing of experience leads to a team approach which includes the patient as a participant.

The nursing service has worked closely with the *laundry and housekeeping services*. Since a fire resistant material had to be used for a uniform and for patient linen, the nursing staff designed a coverall in the same color and material which was selected for patient linen. Maintaining a safe environment is the responsibility of all personnel, especially in this unit. Housekeeping is high on the priority list because the unit is used for both animals (experimental research) and humans. The selection of cleaning solutions must be based on known facts regarding compression and decompression involving the use of oxygen. All volatile substances must be excluded.

The program of *fire prevention* is highest on the priority list of needs. The consequences of a fire in such a confined space are potentially great. When the chamber is pressurized there is no means of immediate escape.

Because of the increased atmospheric pressure, *physics* plays a major role in many aspects of care. Implosion (bursting inward) may occur in the bottles used for intravenous therapy. The use of bags, as for banking blood, may be foreseen in future. The pharmacy staff have done some fine experimentation in the use of drugs as affected by increasing pressures.

The program of *space allocation* has been a major factor. Locker rooms, office space, clean and "dirty" utility rooms, and a staff lounge area were planned. The unit itself is housed in a facility adjoining the semi-private pavilion.

Legal aspects of the project have been considered in terms of personnel health qualifications and waivers, and patient consents and waivers. The need to devise record keeping methods which will be appropriate and practical for the present and for posterity has been a concern. A hyperbaric oxygenation treatment record has become part of the patient's chart. Regulations regarding items for inclusion in the operating room's ledgers were observed. The log was devised as a means of recording information on exposure, current information, and research data (Fig. 5). Utilization of this form assures that certain pertinent areas will be considered when recording the effects of pressurization. Some of the areas which we felt needed to be considered are: (1) physiological and psychological responses, such as dizziness, voice changes, and euphoria; (2) factors which may influence reaction, e.g., lack of sleep or food; (3) objective observation of patients made by the staff outside the chamber or by persons within the chamber.

THE SPECIFIC ROLE OF THE NURSE

The nurse's role to date has been concerned in three areas of preparation and understandings. Medical therapy, surgical procedures, and experimental research call upon the talents of nursing.

The nurse's role in *medical therapy* has been one of progressive learning. There are several points which might be designated as the nurse's responsiblity. The preparation of the chamber is concerned with the functioning of the oxygen and suction systems, the blood pressure apparatus, emergency sets, and the necessary drugs. The availability of special equipment is determined by the individual patient's needs. These needs may include gumdrops, ordering a meal, or an Ambu bag and Bird respirator. Mount Sinai Hospital has made available on a trial basis a stretcher bed made in Zurich, Switzerland, which makes it possible for the patient to be transported everywhere in his bed.

Most patients are admitted to a special area designated for patients receiving hyperbaric oxygenation. Each patient and his family are visited by a member of the nursing staff together with the doctor to explain the chamber and his anticipated experience. Sometimes patients have been too ill for this preparation and so the members of the family are given this support. Some of the important points covered include: the constant availability of staff with the patient in the chamber, so that the patient will never be left alone; the fact that the nurse and doctor experience the same feelings, for example "blocking" of the ear relieved by swallowing, and some pain in the ear which may be uncomfortable but not indicative of any complications; the fact that machinery and noise can be compared to that of an airplane.

When a *surgical* procedure is to take place the nursing staff plans as though an operating room schedule is to be carried out. Organizationally the unit is a part of the operating room, so that the initial planning considered this in terms of instruments, equipment, and supplies. Linens, because of their special preparation, are stored in the unit's area. In essence, the hyperbaric chamber is an additional operating room suite.

The *experimental* work has included oxygen tolerance tests, analysis of blood gases at varying atmospheric pressures, and surgical procedures on dogs.

The hyperbaric nursing staff shares the duties and responsibilities of patient care with the staff of the unit where the patient is located. A nursing care plan is developed for each patient and is maintained cooperatively by the nursing staffs. This plan is used by the nurse who accompanies the patient in the chamber. There is a commitment to insure the continuity of psychological, emotional, and spiritual support.

The nurse applies the face mask to the patient as the pressurization is started and/or as it has been prescribed. The oxygen is adjusted through regulators. During this period a great deal of emotional support is sustained by the nurse. It is the nurse who must be aware of and alert to any signs of untoward reaction to the oxygen, i.e., changes in the respiratory rate, twitching, or any unusual involvement which may be the beginning of convulsions. At the prescribed time decompression is about to be started, the oxygen is discontinued and the mask is removed. This procedure is closely guarded by the hyperbaric technicians who follow the Navy decompression tables. The nurse must be alert to any signs of spontaneous penumothorax or air embolus. Joint pains may be reported by the patient or any of the personnel.

All staff and patients are required to remain in the area for at least an hour after decompression in case any signs of the "bends" should appear. The time is spent with the patient, preparing for the next patient, and recording information on appropriate sheets.

Our experiences have been varied in less than a year. Patients have been treated for gas gangrene, tetanus, anaerobic infections, and arterial insufficiency. A number of patients have had surgical procedures including bilateral sympathectomies and a patch graft to correct a coarctation of the aorta.

The potential of hyperbaric nursing is founded on the medical program and the findings relative to research. Certainly in this day of space and missile programs, the horizons are limitless. Nursing has an innate responsibility to keep pace as our role broadens and expands.

REFERENCES

1. Jensen, J. Trygve, Ed.D.: Introduction to Medical Physics. Philadelphia, J. B. Lippincott Co., 1960.
2. U.S. Navy Diving Manual: Washington, D.C., Bureau of Ships, Navy Department, 1963.
3. Venger, Mary Jane, and Jacobson, J. H.: Nursing plans for a hyperbaric unit. Am. J. Nursing, 64:79, 1964.

Mount Sinai Hospital
100th Street and Fifth Avenue
New York, N.Y. 10029

The Patient and the Bennett

by KAREN H. MCARDLE, B.S.*

The first duty the newborn has in the world is to take the breath of life. Without it he is doomed. One of the last activities we engage in is to breathe our last breath at death. Between these two absolutes of first and last we take our breathing mechanism largely for granted. It is such an unconscious effort that we hardly notice that we breathe at all until misfortune of some type strikes. Then our ability to maintain the breathing process comes to consciousness and becomes of extreme importance.

THE PHYSIOLOGY OF RESPIRATION

Respiration involves moving air in and out of the lungs and the internal exchange of gases with the blood. This frocess is dependent upon the two factors of pressure and concentration. The respiratory substances pass from higher to lower pressures and from higher to lower concentrations. As the thorax and lungs expand, the intrapulmonary pressure decreases. The cartilaginous rings of the trachea and bronchi prevent collapse of these structures and air rushes toward the low pressure area which is within the lungs. Atmospheric air contains about 79.0% nitrogen, 20.9% oxygen and a trace of carbon dioxide. The partial pressure of oxygen is highest in atmospheric air and gradually decreases as it passes through the lungs and into the blood stream. The reverse is true of carbon dioxide; thus oxygen flows from higher concentrations and pressures in the atmosphere to lower ones within the lung.

The lungs expand for several reasons: negative intrapleural and intrapulmonary pressure, surface tension between the pleura, elasticity of the tissue, patency of the airways, and muscular effort to increase the size of the thorax. When there is interference in any of these

---

* Instructor, Misericordia Hospital School of Nursing, Bronx, New York.

areas respiratory distress ensues. It is at this point that machines such as the Bennett respirator prove their usefulness.

INTERMITTENT POSITIVE PRESSURE BREATHING

Use of the intermittent positive pressure breathing (I.P.P.B.) apparatus inflates or assists the lungs during inspiration by positive pressure. Expiration is passive through the release or reduction of pressure to zero; however, in some cases the air can actually be sucked out of the lungs. The unit may be adjusted to cycle automatically or it may be triggered by the patient's own inspiratory effort. A very minimum of effort is required to trigger the Bennett. The controls of the unit are noninteracting; thus operation complexity is avoided.

The I.P.P.B. apparatus may be used in controlled ventilation, in respiratory assistance, and in therapy. Bennett respiration units provide three types of respiratory aid. The first is nonautomatic and patient controlled, and is used in therapy. The second provides cycling and pressure assistance. The automatic cycling rate is set slightly slower than the patient's normal breathing rate to assure respiration if the patient does not breathe voluntarily, and to assist inspiration with positive pressure. Third, the unit may be automatically cycled for controlled ventilation.

EFFECTS OF I.P.P.B.

The purposes or effects of I.P.P.B. may be listed as follows:

1. Without increasing the work of breathing, respiratory insufficiency is relieved or overcome through active inflation of the lungs, deeper and more adequate ventilation, and an increase in the tidal volume.

2. Aerosols are efficiently administered deep into congested, poorly ventilated areas of the lungs, relieving membranous congestion, reducing bronchospasm, and loosening mucous plugs.

3. With more uniform aeration of the alveoli, the respiratory blood gas exchange is improved.

4. A nonfatiguing aid to reeducation for improved breathing habits is provided.

5. Better bronchial drainage is promoted as a result of a high velocity gas flow which occurs when there is a rapid release of the inspiratory pressure during the initial expiratory phase.

6. A more efficient cough mechanism is established by ventilating beyond retained secretions, thus allowing the cough to move them from the area.

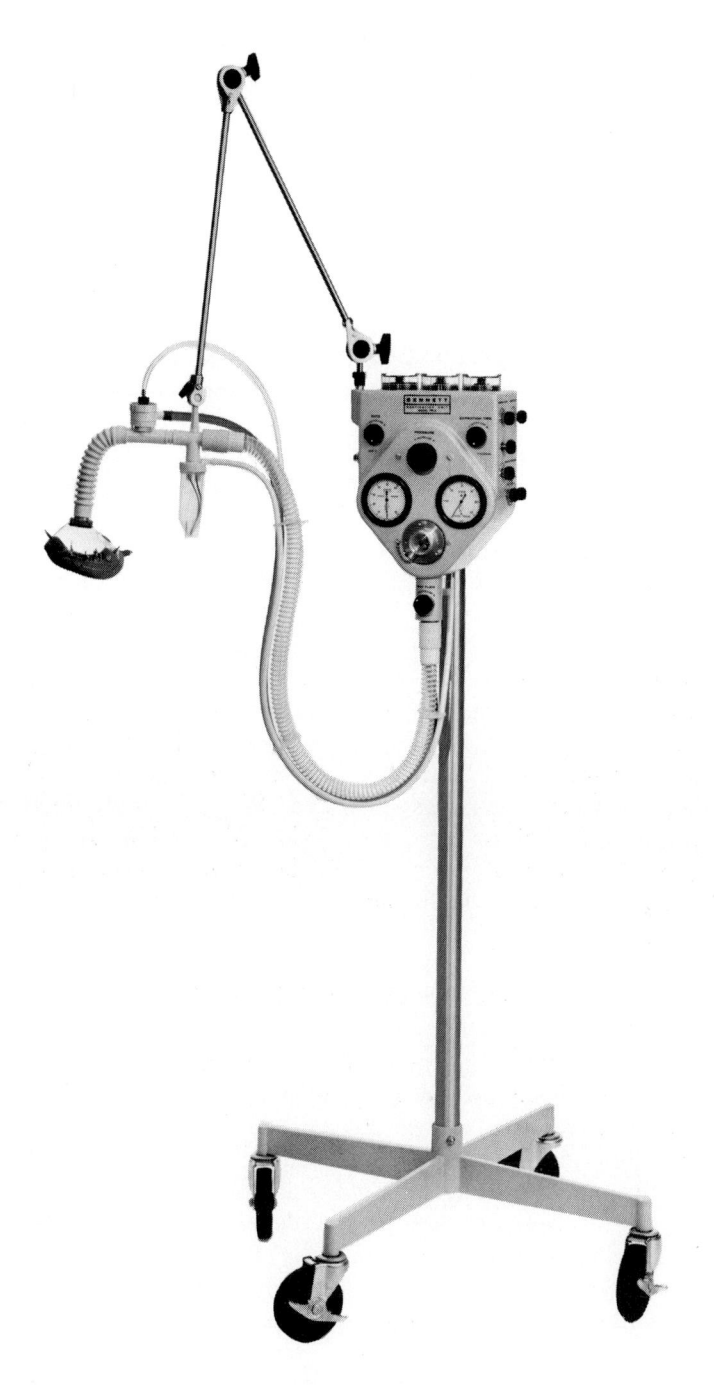

Figure 1. The Bennett respirator.

7. Excess carbon dioxide in the blood is eliminated by washing out alveolar carbon dioxide. This is important in respiratory acidosis.

8. A form of deep breathing exercise is provided which stretches respiratory muscles and seems to enhance the elastic tone and circulation of the lungs.

INDICATIONS FOR I.P.P.B.

Indications for the use of I.P.P.B. include bronchiectasis, asthma, pulmonary fibrosis, acute bronchitis, and pneumonia. The procedure also is used as a prophylactic measure postoperatively, especially after cardiac surgery and valve repairs, and in cases of pulmonary edema and atelectasis. It has nearly abolished the need for tank respirators, and can be used in respiratory arrest or paralysis, respiratory acidosis, some intoxications, and with airway obstructions due to secretions, mucosal edema, or alveolar exudate.

Medications may be administered as aerosols by the Bennett apparatus and serve a combination of purposes. Bronchodilators such as Isuprel and Vaponefrin may be used to relieve bronchospasm. They should be diluted prior to administration and Isuprel should never be used if it contains a precipitate or has become brown in color. Antibiotic drugs such as tetracycline and penicillin may be employed in infectious processes. Surface tension reducers, detergents, and mucolytic agents such as Alevaire and Mucomyst soften secretions and make them less tenacious, thus more easily expectorated. Water is used effectively for the humidification of inspired air. If heated humidification is being employed, the use of Alevaire should be avoided because it leaves a tenacious deposit in the flow valve.

OPERATION OF THE RESPIRATOR

To use the machine the nurse should become acquainted with the literature the company provides; however, a few general rules of operation can be stated here. These rules generally apply whether the machine is being used for therapy, assistance, or control.

1. The machine must be connected to a source of oxygen or whatever type of gaseous mixture has been ordered. The connection will be found on the back of the unit.

2. The pressure control gauge is turned to the right until the Control Pressure dial shows the desired pressure as prescribed by the physician. With adults the initial pressure used varies from 10 to 20 cm. H_2O. For use of the unit in a pediatric service the initial pressure will understandably be lower. (See Figure 2.)

3. The Dilution control is set for the prescribed oxygen concentration by pushing the knob all the way in for 40% and pulling it all the way out for 100% concentration. Concentration between these figures is estimated.

4. The prescribed medication is put into the nebulizer vial or distilled water is used if no other humidification is provided. The nebulization controls are adjusted for inspiration only or for continuous nebulization.

5. If the machine is being used for control of the patient's respiration the Rate control is set for automatic cycling. If the patient is breathing on his own but his breathing is weak or erratic, the control is set slightly slower than his rate. This can be determined by listening to the sound of the machine. Inspiration and expiration are clearly distinguished.

6. Other controls are set at "Off" or "Normal" unless ordered by the physician.

NURSING RESPONSIBILITIES WITH THE I.P.P.B

Once the machine has been set up, nursing care involves four major areas of responsibility. The *first* is the avoidance or control of as many leaks as possible. Preparations should be made for this purpose before the machine is started. If a face mask is being used, facial oils should be removed as completely as possible. If the cushion around the edge of the mask is not completely inflated, opening the valve at the bottom of the cushion allows the self-filling device to re-inflate it.

If tracheostomy or endotracheal tubes are being used, they should be cuffed; that is, a seal should be maintained around the orifice where the tube enters. If a mouthpiece is being used, the patient should be instructed to bite down gently on it and to seal his lips around it. The patient should understand that he must breathe entirely through his mouth when using the mouthpiece.

The Bennett respirator functions in spite of gross air leaks; however, efficiency increases in inverse proportion to air leakage. Tubing and all parts of the apparatus should be securely connected. At each inspiration the System Pressure and Control Pressure readings on the front dials should be similar.

The *second* area of nursing responsibility is to keep a continual check on the machine itself, and this is done by observation and thoughtful listening. The patient may be in a sitting or a recumbent position when using the machine. Once use of the machine has begun, the nurse listens for its regular rhythmic cycle. Observing the regular movement of the three pistons on the top of the unit also is a good indication that the automatic cycling mechanism is functioning properly.

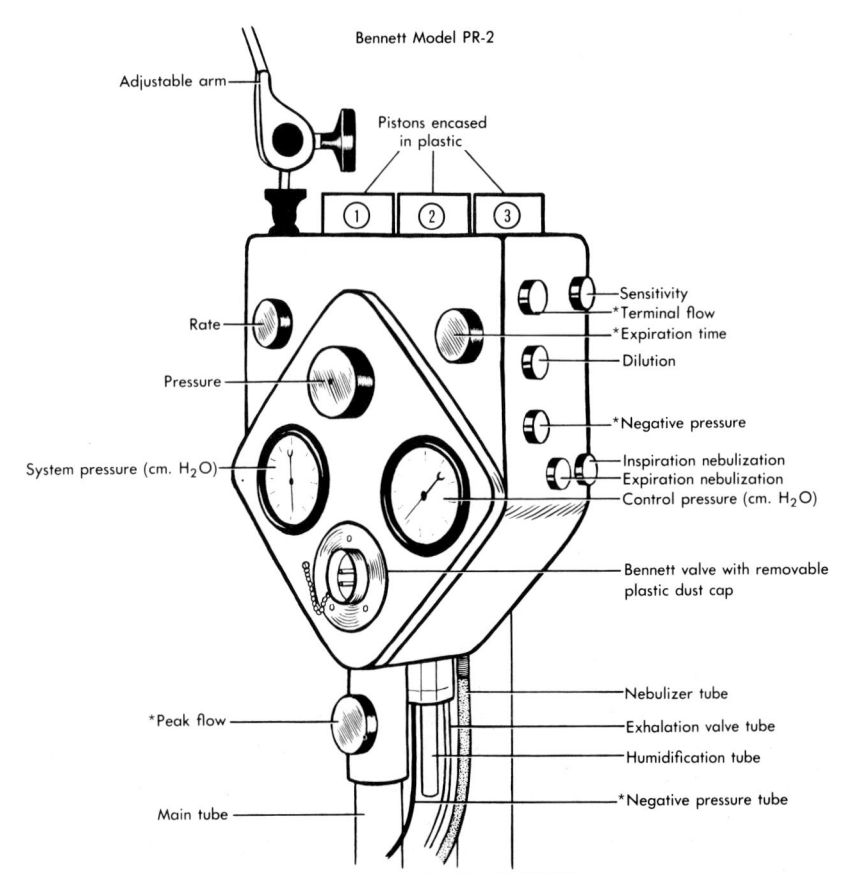

Figure 2. Adjustable arm: This supports the various tubes, the nebulizer, and the face mask, mouth piece or tracheostomy attachment. Pistons: The first piston (1) controls the length of expiration time. The second (2) rephases the other pistons and the third (3) controls the length of inspiration time. Sensitivity: This control alollows a feeble inspiratory effort by the patient to trigger the machine. It is adjustable for negative inspiratory impulses of less than 1.5 cm. H_2O. Terminal flow: This is the flow at which the valve closes, and with the Model PR-2 is less than 1 LPM (liter per minute). It is the flow at the end of inspiration and the minimum flow at which the valve will open and remain open until control pressure is reached. This adjustor helps prevent premature cycling and helps to compensate for leaks or low flow from the nebulizer. Rate: The Rate control sets automatic cycling from 0–50 cycles per minute and can control the automatic start of inspiration and expiration. Expiration time: This control modifies the rate setting to increase the length of expiration time while inspiration remains fixed. When the control is set in the "Normal" position and the Rate control is turned on, the breathing cycle is established at a 1 to $1\frac{1}{2}$ ratio of inspiration to expiration—for example, a 2 second inspiration and a 3 second expiration. The rate does not affect the ratio. The ratio may be adjusted to 1 to 2, 1 to 3 or more with the Expiration Time control. Dilution: Oxygen concentrations may be given from 40% (knob pushed all the way in) up to 100% (knob pulled all the way out). Dilutions may be changed without

PATIENT OBSERVATION DURING USE OF THE MACHINE

The *third* area of responsibility is observation of the patient. If the patient is using the machine for long periods of time or is being controlled by it, hyperventilation may occur. As a result the carbon dioxide is being removed at a rapid rate, the pH of the arterial blood increases, and respiratory alkalosis ensues. Symptoms may include head or chest pain, tingling or numbness in the fingers and toes, vertigo, syncope, and, in extreme states, carpopedal spasms and other signs of tetany. Complications may be avoided by slowing the respiratory rate. It must be remembered also that the patient's desire or need to breathe decreases as the oxygen concentration of the blood increases. The syndrome may arise more quickly in children than with adults.

If the patient is in a coma or is unconscious and is being maintained or controlled by the machine, the nurse should check for gastric distention. Occasionally the epiglottis may fall over the larynx allowing air to escape into the stomach. Using a cuffed tracheostomy or endotracheal tube obviates the hazard. Again, the signs of cyanosis and gastric distention appear more quickly in the child than in the adult. If the

---

altering the other controls. A sintered bronze filter found on the opposite side panel removes dust and lint from the air and can be taken apart for easy cleaning. Pressure: This sets the control pressure by turning the dial to the right. Negative pressure: This control sets negative expiration pressure and is used primarily to augment filling of the right heart or for immediate handling of an upper airway obstruction. The pressure is adjustable from 0–6 cm. H_2O. System pressure: The pressure is measured in cm. H_2O and the dial indicates the pressure in the tube system and at the mouth. It does not give the pressure in the lungs. Inspiration nebulization: This controls medications or humidity in the inspired gas. Expiration nebulization: This controls medications or humidity in the manifold and tube for initial inspiratory flow. It allows for continuous nebulization. Control pressure: This is also measured in cm. H_2O and indicates the pressure that will be reached in the tube system if inspiration is pressure limited, i.e., nonautomatic cycling. Bennett valve: The valve opens in response to slight inspiratory effort, allows a variable flow, then closes when the flow diminishes to a low terminal point. The unit cycles automatically if the patient stops breathing or if his respiration drops below the set rate. While on automatic operation the patient can override the machine and breathe his own pattern without mechanical interference. The machine works with the patient, not the patient with the machine. Nebulizer tube: The tube connects with the nebulizer found at the distal base of the adjustable arm of the unit. Peak flow: This control adjusts the maximum peak flow from the Bennett valve and thus is able to limit the flow the unit can deliver. It allows for slower filling of the lungs and a more gradual than usual rise to control pressure. Exhalation valve tube: This relieves waste gases. Humidfication tube: This is connected to a humidifier found below the unit. Humidification may be accomplished with room temperature solutions or they may be heated by means of a special device which is inserted directly into the solution. Negative pressure tube: This tube is connected and used only when negative pressure is ordered by the physician. Main tube: This is the primary tube through which the bulk of the gases, medications and humidity pass.

condition does occur, gastric suction may be used to relieve the stomach of air.

Concluding that ventilation is adequate for the patient is done after watching the expansion of the chest on inspiration, checking his color, feeling a normal pulse, and observing the System Pressure gauge. The latter will give an estimate of how much pressure is entering at the mouth or trachea. The Control Pressure gauge is not an accurate check. If hidden leaks are present, part of the pressure will be used to supply the leak and this will not be detected by the Control Pressure gauge.

If oxygen is being given through a tracheostomy postoperatively, it is important that the patient be positioned to provide ease of breathing and to facilitate the removal of secretions. Breath sounds can be checked with a stethoscope, and gentle suction should be employed as necessary.

When the respirator is used for periods of 30 minutes or more at a pressure of 20 cm. H_2O or above with the adult patient, filling of the right heart may be impaired. This complication could conceivably occur in children at a lower pressure. A reduction in pulse volume on inspiration is an early indication of this problem. Lengthening the expiration phase may obviate or control the situation.

The air passages should not be allowed to dry up. If the unit is being used for long periods some type of humidification should be employed. On the other hand, if surface tension reducers or wetting agents are being administered, secretions should be expectorated or suctioned off as soon as it is safely possible.

If the patient is receiving bronchodilators the nurse should observe for overdosage or excessive nebulization flow rate. Palpitations or nervousness may indicate that this has occurred. In pediatrics the critical acumen of the nurse will probably be the best guarantee of the patient's safety. Because children are not so inhibited from acting exactly as they feel, their activity sets up guidelines for the nurse's observations.

The area of communication is involved here. Not only are children unable to express in words much of the information the nurse needs to know, but any patient, whether child or adult, is unable to speak while using the Bennett. It is important for the nurse to get to know the patient as well as possible as soon as possible so that she may be that much better prepared to anticipate his needs.

Fear is often present when the machine is being used, and the mere continual presence of the nurse may do much to allay anxiety.

THE TEACHING FUNCTION OF THE NURSE

If the Bennett is to be used postoperatively it is best to introduce and demonstrate it and have the patient use it preoperatively. In pediatrics the unit has been used with postoperative cardiac patients, and it may also be used to administer oxygen following surgery.

This brings us to the last area of responsibility for nursing a patient using a Bennett respirator. That area is teaching. The nurse teaches the patient how the machine operates, how to use it, and how to cough effectively, that is, to bring up deep secretions before and after each treatment. All available powers of creativity will come into play when teaching the child about the unit. The face mask and the noise of the machine are probably the most common elements causing fear in the child. If the nurse can make a game of it by trying it on herself first, the child may not be as reluctant to try and may find the treatment more acceptable. For example, the nurse sets the scene in a Gemini space capsule. She puts on the face mask before the rocket blasts off. A big sound from the rocket (Bennett) is made and a great rush of air comes through the mask so the astronaut (patient) can breathe well while he is in space. The amount of information and story-telling the child is given depends upon his age, level of understanding, and degree of excitability.

If oxygen is being given through a tracheostomy postoperatively it is important that the nurse position the patient for ease of breathing and to facilitate the removal of secretions. Breath sounds can be checked with a stethoscope and gentle suction should be employed as necessary.

When the respirator is used at intervals lasting 30 minutes or more using 20 cm. H_2O or above with the adult patient, filling of the right heart may be impaired. This complication could conceivably occur in children also with less pressure being used. A reduction in pulse volume on inspiration is an early indication of this problem. Lengthening the expiration phase may obviate or control the situation.

SUMMARY

To recapitulate, the four major areas of nursing responsibility in use of the Bennett respirator are preventing or controlling air leakage, keeping a continual check on the machine, maintaining constant observation of the patient, and patient teaching. Good performance in all areas is necessary for the patient's welfare and safety and none of the areas can be listed as more or less important than the next if the patient and the Bennett are to reach the maximum potential intended.

THE FIRST HOME VISIT

The nurse, in visiting the home, attempts to form an objective picture of how and where the child fits into the family constellation. His position in the family will be an important factor in his adjustment to his return home and his rehabilitation.

The equipment or supplies needed for the child's care should be ascertained and provision made for acquiring them if they are not already available. Equipment already in the home is utilized whenever possible. Through discussion and exploration with the family adaptations can often be made.

Another very important aspect of the first visit is identifying areas that lend themselves to self-help activities, such as the bathroom utilities. Is it possible for the child to reach the sink or will a stool or box be needed for his use? Is it reasonable to expect that the child can get in and out of bed with the present furniture or will an overhead bar or trapeze be needed? Observations of this type will help the nurse in future planning. It may take many conferences with the parents to discover ways of making the home easier for the child to be self-sufficient.

The nurse identifies tasks that will be carried out for the child. The ultimate aim is to have the child assume as much responsibility for these as possible. However, at first it may be necessary to have other members of the household perform some of them. If the family has not already delegated these responsibilities, the nurse can help them work out a plan. It is a mistake to assume that the parents always will do this. Many times other children in the home can be made to feel important if they are included in the plans. It may be necessary for the nurse herself to be responsible for some of the more difficult tasks. Each child presents a different picture, and the plan must be specifically designed for him.

With the current emphasis on the high cost of medical care it is perhaps superfluous to remind the nurse to check on the financial strain of this illness. However, long-term illness has some unique features and one is the ability to cause a financial strain at any time. Hospital insurance often has satisfactorily covered inpatient care but now the child will be carried as an outpatient, very likely without insurance coverage.

This may seem to call for a lengthy first visit, and usually that is the case. The groundwork laid here will be of utmost value for future visits and time should not be a factor. Assume before you make this visit that its duration will have to be flexible because of the many unknown factors which will present themselves.

FIRST INTERVIEW WITH THE CHILD

The child is a member of his family and as much as possible should be treated within this context. A separate interview with him is necessary specifically to find out how the child is reacting to his illness. His self-image may have been severely affected by an illness of this degree. He may need to talk through what this illness means to him.

Only the child can give you a clear picture of the best way to help him achieve maximum independence. A plan of rehabilitation is useless if the child has decided he likes the role of dependence and finds it very comfortable. A first interview may not supply any information but you may start to gain the child's confidence.

DEALING WITH THE EFFECTS OF HOSPITALIZATION

The nurse needs to be alert for signs of the effects of hospitalization on the child, immediate or delayed. Early manifestations may be clinging to the parents and not wanting mother to be out of sight. A conference with the mother may make this stage easier to accept. Parents who know that this is a normal reaction are less likely to become overly concerned. The assurance that with proper handling and time this reaction will pass gives the parents a feeling of relief. After some of these temporary reactions have passed, the long-term illness is easier to accept and work around.

The nurse is in an excellent position to evaluate the severity of these reactions to hospitalization and to intervene when necessary. For instance, if a child has regressed in eating to the point that he wants to be fed instead of feeding himself, the nurse can outline steps the mother can take to overcome this. For example, explain to the child that he must feed himself. Then place the food attractively and conveniently in front of him. Provide adequate utensils and a friendly warm atmosphere. Be sure the child rests before the meal and then comes to the table.

The child is given adequate time, considering his age and handicap, to eat. At the end of this time the plate is removed and the child is excused from the table. The amount of food he has consumed does not determine the length of time. No provision is made for snacking. No emphasis is put on poor performance. Praise is given only if earned. Consistency is one of the prime factors in such a program and will certainly influence the results.

PREVENTIVE INTERVENTION BY THE PUBLIC HEALTH NURSE

The public health nurse attempts to prevent undesirable occurrences by working with the child and his surroundings. For example, in the case of a child with a new hearing aid, the nurse has the child demonstrate how he takes out and inserts the ear piece. She also suggests that the child demonstrate this in "show and tell" sessions at school. She may ask the teacher to talk to the class about hearing aids and how delicate they are. If the mystery is taken out of the aid the children no longer feel the need to explore on their own. They also learn that the cord does not get pulled to attract the child's attention.

Another possibility for preventive intervention is in relation to nutrition for the newly paralyzed child. Before the child learns to walk with crutches and braces he often is confined to a wheel chair. His sudden decrease in activity will call for a decrease in food intake. A well planned, nutritious diet with decreased amount of calories and fat is indicated. It is harder to lose weight than to control weight gain, and an overweight child is hampered in learning to walk.

The handicapped person usually is more likely to develop secondary urinary infections and respiratory infections than the normal person, and the nursing care plan for the handicapped child must of necessity include means of preventing, or coping with, such complications.

There are many other areas which call for preventive intervention, and the creative nurse will try to look into the future and anticipate the possibilities that lie ahead.

THE IMPORTANCE OF FOLLOW-UP APPOINTMENTS

The role of follow-up cannot receive too much emphasis when working with the handicapped child. The parents may become discouraged by the many follow-up appointments, especially when the child is feeling well. It is easier for them to see the need for appointments which help provide a cure.

The public health nurse holds a key role in teaching the family the value of keeping appointments. Occasionally communications break down between the family and the doctor or institution caring for the child. When this happens the nurse can intervene and see that communications are reestablished.

Follow-up includes more than medical supervision. The child has to be integrated back into school, church, peer groups and the like. It may be necessary to contact the school nurse about adaptations needed in order for the child to attend school successfully. The public health nurse does not assume total responsibility for this type of follow-up but she should not sit back and assume that someone else will do it, either.

EXAMPLES OF HANDICAPPING CONDITIONS IN VARIOUS AGE GROUPS

1. *John Jones—a baby with a congenital absence of the left upper extremity.*

The baby born with a missing extremity is a shock and disappointment to his parents. During the hospital period Mrs. Jones may have had an opportunity to work through some of her feelings regarding her handicapped baby. On the first home visit the public health nurse gives Mrs. Jones a chance to talk about John. In addition, she observes the way Mrs. Jones handles her baby. The simplest observations may be important. For example, how close does she hold him? What does she call him? How is he dressed? Where was the baby when the nurse arrived? Does it appear that John is being hidden away?

During the visit the nurse cuddles John and handles him with respect. She demonstrates by her acceptance of the baby that he is a fine baby. Her reaction to John may be the only positive reaction the mother has seen since her return home from the hospital. Unfortunately, curious friends and relatives may have come just to view the defect rather than John.

It is important not to concentrate the whole visit around the handicap. In the hospital Mrs. Jones may not have been ready to learn how to bathe John or to make his formula. She may need encouragement to get started back on the road to normal living.

It is a poor policy to assume that Mrs. Jones will be immobilized by the situation. She may be driven to do more than she should, at this time, to keep her mind off the baby. Mrs. Jones might very well respond to some real concern about how well she feels. It sometimes happens that in our enthusiasm to do the very best for the handicapped child we neglect to give the proper supervision to our postpartum patient.

As John grows, new situations present themselves. The public health nurse is able to encourage Mrs. Jones in acceptance of the prosthesis. Each institution or rehabilitation center has its own rationale for the correct time to fit the child with a prosthesis. Mrs. Jones may find the idea of a prosthesis with a hook repugnant. She may have imagined an artificial hand and may be very disappointed when she finds out the child will not have one. A fine pamphlet on prostheses by the Children's Bureau[2] can be a marvelous aid in helping Mrs. Jones over this hump.

The need for the prosthesis will be very well demonstrated to Mrs. Jones when John attempts to crawl, without success. John will also be frustrated when he tries to play with toys. He will be the biggest help in getting Mrs. Jones to accept the prosthesis after he is fitted, since it soon becomes very apparent that John can do many new things with it.

Care specific to the prosthesis is covered with the family. The nurse points out the necessity of keeping it clean and free of dust, and checking the straps and areas which may cause irritation. She also encourages its continual use.

2. *Ann Marie is a toddler with cystic fibrosis.*

The toddler with a long-term illness is really a challenge to the nurse. It is important to keep in mind the normal developmental facts relevant to this age group when planning nursing care. These include his task of establishing autonomy, the power of magical thought, his tendency to have temper tantrums, his masturbation to relieve tension, his tendency to get into everything, his thumbsucking, his fear of losing his parents' love, his need to have limits set, his ambivalence about toilet training, the fact that he understands language much better than he can use it, his clinging to a favorite toy, and his engaging in parallel play.

An important part of the home care will be getting Ann Marie to accept *medications*. It is wisest to let her know she is getting medication. However, if she prefers it in juice or followed by fruit, this is acceptable. It is also important to keep medications marked correctly and stored high up where the child cannot help herself to an overdose. Although she may put up a fuss when given medications on time, she may take them willingly if she finds the bottle as part of her own exploration.

Postural drainage is another area in which the nurse can offer suggestions and supervision. If the family is using a drainage board the techniques may be the same as those used in the hospital. However, if a board is not available the public health nurse can demonstrate placing the toddler over her knee in a comfortable position. This can be done as a game and the toddler will cooperate. You may need to demonstrate using an older child at first, as the toddler fears being dropped. During the cupping procedure, you can make up a song such as "tap tap on Ann Marie." The words are not as important as the rhythm and repetition.

Inhalation therapy may be ordered in the home. In this day and age the mask can be imagined as almost anything related to science. Children's TV shows will give you all kinds of ideas for making this a perfectly acceptable game. At night when the child is in a tent it can be his space house or his air conditioner.

Another area of major concern to Ann Marie is *nutrition*. Frequent feedings are needed to assure adequate assimilation of food. Fancy dishes, straws if she has mastered the technique, paper plates to suggest a picnic, a relaxing atmosphere with records, appropriate sized furniture, and small helpings with an opportunity for "seconds" are all helpful. Normal dietary requirements are to be followed, with emphasis on protein and lowered fat intake. In the summer additional salt is indicated.

Encouraging normal activity to help prevent stasis of the thick secretions is indicated.

Again the role of the nurse in supporting the parents cannot be overemphasized. Cystic fibrosis has been advertised everywhere as a "killer of children." With this publicity the parents tend to overprotect their child. The life expectancy for these children has increased significantly and it is important to prepare them for a long life. The parents may also ask about having more children. Despite the nurse's knowledge of the incidence of this disease, it is important that the parents get good genetic counseling and the nurse should refer the parents to an appropriate source.[4] After the initial counseling, the nurse is in an excellent position to clarify and emphasize what the physician has said.

3. *Jimmy is a preschooler with cerebral palsy.*

Cerebral palsy today has an increasing incidence with our increasing ability to save precarious pregnancies and to save the lives of more premature babies.

Jimmy has recently been hospitalized for a heel cord lengthening and is returning home. He has bilateral casts on his legs. The usual cast care is demonstrated to the parents, including cleaning of the cast, checking the circulation of toes, and looking for foreign objects that Jimmy may put in his cast.

The normal growth and developmental pattern will be altered, depending on the type and severity of the cerebral palsy. If Jimmy has normal intelligence, he should be working on establishing initiative. He has already mastered trust and autonomy, so both of these can be utilized in his care. He also has the power of magical thought and a vivid imagination. He has an interest and anxiety about sex differences. He is curious about everything and he begins to develop a conscience. His motor skills are increasing as well as his vocabulary.

It is quite evident that being in a cast is interfering with Jimmy's normal development. His aims will have to be to use his upper extremities to compensate for his motor impairment. This may be a real problem if he does not have control of his arms and hands.

Utensils for feeding may have to be especially made for him. He may have to have toys that are weighted on the bottom or books with heavy pages that he can turn himself.

If his speech is affected, it may be necessary to listen attentively and encourage Jimmy to want to communicate verbally. An adult who becomes frustrated trying to understand the child readily conveys this impression to the child, and he gives up attempts. If speech is out of the question, a well designed pantomime communication may be used. As the child gets older, writing or typing also will be attempted.

The preschooler will need continual reassurance that his legs are still there, hidden by the casts. In addition, the parents need to be alerted to the fact that the child will interpret the casts as part of himself, so that he will need preparation for their removal.

Nutritional requirements will depend on the type of cerebral palsy, with the additional consideration of decreased locomotion due to the casts.

Other factors that will influence the nursing care are whether or not Jimmy has been taught crutch walking and whether or not he has walking calipers on his cast. Jimmy should not be allowed to regress on account of his surgery, and the nurse should encourage ambulation, if this is possible.

Regression in toilet training may result from the hospitalization. Jimmy's wooden potty chair may be easier to use than the toilet. It may be necessary to have a urinal available while he is in bed. A glass jar or tin can may be painted gaily for this purpose.

A pet can be a marvelous companion for the immobilized child. Animals such as goldfish, turtles or a bird are inexpensive but priceless in value.

4. *Loretta is a school-age child with rheumatic fever.*

The most difficult stage of rheumatic fever is the long convalescent period when the child is feeling well.

The school-age child is in the period of industry, from six to twelve years. There is a need of peer relationships and to be active in clubs. A gnawing desire exists to learn and to explore his environment. The love of competition in sports and school work is developing.

Loretta will be deprived of many of these activities because of the nature of her illness. Bed rest may be extremely taxing to her and her family. It is easy to say that the nurse should teach the importance of bed rest, but to a child, with her short attention span, her innate burning desire to be on the go and her need to break away from her home, this is easier said than done.

Ways of making bed rest more tolerable are to place the bed near a window so she can watch outside activity, to give her a cheerful room of her own, and to provide many outside interests. The hand-eye coordination has now been developed so reading is a good pastime, as are sewing, knitting and weaving. Scheduled visits of peers can include games of checkers, cards or Monopoly. Judicious use of TV can be included in the daily activities. Pretty pajamas, hair ribbons or jewelry provide a change of pace. School work should be provided by either a home teacher or a take-home service from school.

The school-age child has an awareness of death and any illness that affects her heart may be particularly frightening to her. She will want simple and continual explanations of her illness and how she is progressing. Her anxieties may also include falling behind in school and the expense of this illness to her family.

The personal hygiene of the school-age child usually leaves something to be desired. Loretta may need encouragement to bathe daily despite her confinement to bed. She will probably have her permanent teeth, and it is extremely important to keep them free of caries. She will need to know that when dental extractions are necessary, she must notify the dentist of her illness so he can give her extra antibiotics.

It is an ideal time to teach Loretta about precautions in the future. She is able to understand the need for long-term antibiotics if explained in terms she is familiar with. She should also be taught to seek early attention for upper respiratory conditions, to get adequate rest and to eat a well balanced diet.

5. *Joan is an adolescent who is mentally retarded.*

The normal developmental tasks of this age group will be altered in Joan's case by her mental age and her retarded development. Tasks of her mental age group will be integrated with appropriate tasks of the adolescent. Changes in body shape, size and organs will probably take place, so that good body hygiene and instruction on menstruation are indicated. The food fads of adolescence may be present. Joan may have the normal sex drives so she must understand such simple things as not to get into cars with strangers.

The adolescent also wants to know where he fits into our society. Although Joan may not question, this, appropriate vocational training is indicated and the public health nurse can be instrumental in making the appropriate referral.

Social contacts are very necessary for Joan. She will benefit from contacts with other mentally retarded persons as well as with normal children. She is encouraged to try new things which will stimulate learning even if a certain amount of frustration ensues. Joan must learn that all experiences are not satisfying.

SUMMARY

Suggestions have been given as to how the public health nurse can work effectively to return the handicapped child to the community after hospitalization. The techniques suggested may be used for many different health problems. Knowledge of the developmental tasks of the particular age period is essential for planning and carrying out nursing care plans; these are altered to meet the needs of the retarded.

REFERENCES

1. Bowman, Peter, and Mautner, Hans, Eds.: Mental Retardation. New York, Grune and Stratton, 1960.
2. The Child with a Missing Arm or Leg. Children's Bureau Folder No. 49-1959, U.S. Goverment Printing Office, Washington 25, D.C.
3. Fishbein, Morris, Ed.: Birth Defects. Philadelphia, J.B. Lippincott Co., 1963.
4. Reed, S.C.: Counseling in Medical Genetics. 2nd Ed. Philadelphia, W.B. Saunders Co., 1963.

69 Bidwell Parkway
Buffalo, New York 14222

Special Features

AN EMINENT PERSONALITY IN NURSING
    Lucile Petry Leone

A PROBLEM IN INTERPERSONAL RELATIONS
    Telling the Truth to Leukemic Children

THE WAY IT WAS
    Leeching

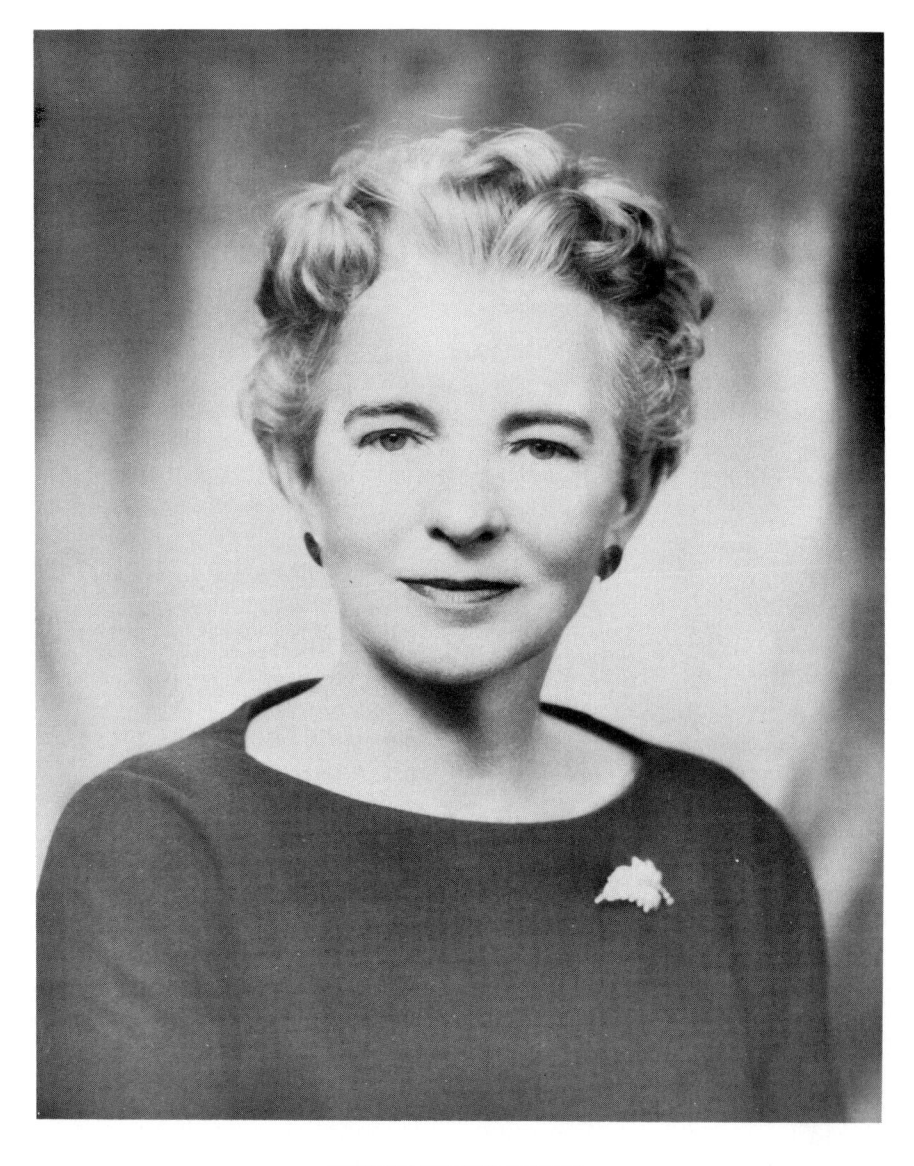

LUCILE PETRY LEONE

An Eminent Personality in Nursing

LUCILE PETRY LEONE

The daughter of a teacher in a one-room country school, Lucile Petry Leone was to become the first Chief Nurse Officer of the Public Health Service and the only woman in the country who answers to the title, "Admiral."

This attractive, petite, blue-eyed woman with an engaging smile was born in Lewisburg, Ohio, but her family later moved to a small town in Delaware where her father became a school principal. It was in this school that she received all of her schooling, being taught Latin and algebra by her father in high school.

She started college without knowing what she was going to do afterwards. It was during her summer vacation at the end of her junior year that she decided she wanted to become a nurse and got a $25.00 a month job as a nurse's aide in a lower East Side hospital in New York. Three days after graduating from college, she entered the Johns Hopkins Hospital School of Nursing.

After receiving her R.N., she became a head nurse in a psychiatric ward where, by accepting $5.00 a month less salary and attending a few classes and conferences, she received a certificate for having completed a postgraduate course in psychiatric nursing. She received the scholarship awarded each year to a graduating senior and went on to obtain her master's degree in supervision from Teachers College, Columbia University. Upon completion of her master's degree, she accepted a position as Supervisor of Clinical Instruction at the School of Nursing, University of Minnesota.

While in Seattle as an Exchange Professor at the University of Washington, Mrs. Leone received a call asking her to come to Washington to be interviewed for a new position in the United States Public Health Service. She accepted the position and began work in the fall of 1941. With two other nurses, she planned a program of Federal aid to nursing education which provided scholarships for young women wishing to become nurses but who needed financial assistance. Shortly after the program began, the United States entered World War II and the program which had been planned was not sufficient to meet the needs. Thus, in July 1943, the U. S. Cadet Nurse Corps was initiated and she became its Director.

The scope of her activities in the Public Health Service has reached every facet of nursing. She was Technical Advisor to the U.S. Delegation at the First and Ninth World Health Assemblies in Geneva and helped to write two of the first nursing publications of the World Health Organization. She has continued her interest in international affairs by calling international seminars, by participating in international meetings, and by extensive personal contact and professional correspondence with nurses all ovr the world.

She has built in the Public Health Service a well trained corps of nurses, including nurses for leadership in all fields of the profession, and she has been a leading influence in nursing research. She has worked toward a better understanding of nurses' roles in health through scores of public addresses and professional papers published in nursing and related journals. She has aided hospitals all over the country in the effective utilization of nursing personnel through counseling and through courses which she gives to students of hospital administration. She has also played a major role in creating public understanding of the national need for more nurses who are educated for the complex tasks of today and the more complex tasks of tomorrow.

All through her career, Mrs. Leone has devoted her energies to furthering nursing education. She has visited schools all over the country, has counseled teachers, deans, and college presidents, and has served on committees conducting special studies of curricula.

In addition to serving two terms (1959–63) as President of the National League for Nursing, she is a member of a number of committees and boards. She has received honorary doctoral degrees from eight universities and has been recipient of many awards, including the American Legion Auxiliary Award, the Florence Nightingale Medal, the Lasker Award to Nursing Services of the Public Health Service, and the Annie Jump Cannon Centennial Medal.

On the occasion of Mrs. Leone's retirement from the United States Public Health Service, all those in nursing and the allied professions unite in according her the traditional "Well done" and in offering her best wishes for a happy future.

A Problem in Interpersonal Relations

TELLING THE TRUTH TO LEUKEMIC CHILDREN
Abridged From Medical World News, September 3, 1965

Nurses will be greatly interested in a program now under way at the National Cancer Institute to help children face the problems of critical illness, hospitalization, and death. Dr. Myron R. Karon, chief pediatrician at the Institute's medical branch, and Joel Vernick of the social service department use any aspect of the hospital environment as a starting point to help their young patients deal with these problems.

When death occurs, every child knows of it, says Dr. Karon. "These hospital-wise children quickly learn to interpret the meaning of the sudden absence of a playmate, the removal of the oxygen tent, the missing nameplate, the room change in the middle of the night."

When the children asked, "What happened to Johnny?" staff members used to answer, "Oh, he went home," or "He went to the 13th floor." Apparently the lies were accepted. How well the children knew the truth, however, became clear when they tried to transfer one 9-year-old to the 13th floor.

Transfer was necessary because of limited space on the leukemia ward, but the child became unmanageable; he was so furious and frightened that he had to be held to protect himself and others. It took more than an hour to find out why. "That's where the kids go to die," he explained. "When kids get sent to the 13th floor, I never see them again."

After that, the staff decided that only the truth is a proper answer to the question of what happened to Johnny. The desire to protect a child from knowledge of death may really be a desire to protect ourselves, the NCI workers believe. And when certain subjects are taboo, too painful for the adult to talk about, the child also becomes mute. Though he "accepts" adult lies, he feels left to cope with his fears and anxieties alone, when he needs adult strength most.

If we really want to help the very sick child face his situation, Mr. Vernick says, "we must develop an environment in which he feels perfectly safe in asking any question and completely confident of receiving an honest answer."

In the past year and a half, 51 patients from 9 to 20 years old have been encouraged to talk with any staff member about their most serious problems. "Any subject, from the pain of a finger prick to the death of a roommate, is fair for discussion," Dr. Karon says, "and any time... is a good time for discussion."

Once a week, the medical staff hold a session with ward nurses to discuss current or future ward problems. Often these meetings bring into the open feelings about illness, hospitalization, death.

Parents of children currently on the ward also meet once a week with Dr. Karon and a medical social worker. Though ostensibly a conference about medical matters, these "group sessions" almost always end with a discussion of such problems as what to tell one's child about leukemia.

The chief aim of the program is to enable the children to live and function well outside the hospital.

There is a clear recognition that, at least by the age of 9 and sometimes earlier, these patients are frightened by their prolonged, severe, and ultimately fatal illness. Therefore, patients are told why procedures are carried out, and they are told their diagnosis as soon as possible.

Older children, especially, are upset when procedures are done without explanation. Said one 14-year-old girl about her liver biopsy, "It's my liver. What am I, some sort of rat or something?"

The first staff member to see a child after the death of another patient says something like this to him: "Johnny died last night. He was very sick." Usually the patient will say, "I knew, but thanks for telling me." Dr. Karon and Mr. Vernick believe this conversation lets the child know he is not as sick as his friend was before he died, and also lets him know that the adults can talk with him. In the experience of the NCI workers, "every child who is lying in bed gravely ill is worrying about dying and is eager to have someone help him talk about it."

Does the program work? Can staff members really help by answering questions honestly and encouraging children to talk about their deepest concerns? Of the 51 patients, "everyone was able to function normally," according to Dr. Karon. "The withdrawal and depression so often observed by others ... occurred very infrequently and were always transient."

Discussion about diagnosis varies with the age and background of the child. The chronic nature of leukemia is indicated, but the children are assured that they will be able to resume normal activities between hospitalizations.

Ideally, parents tell the child his diagnosis. Once the parents know, there is an immediate and inevitable change in their attitude toward the child, which confirms his worst suspicions and deepens his anxieties. If parents cannot bring themselves to tell the child about his condition, they are urged to permit the doctor to do so. Secrecy, the Bethesda workers are convinced, is always more frightening to the youngster than the truth.

They cite an 11-year-old girl who told her mother, "I know there is no cure for leukemia, but at least I'm glad you told me what I have." Before she knew, she said, her mind was going "a mile a minute" thinking about what she might have.

Withholding the diagnosis may contribute to severe behavior problems. A 10-year-old boy was apprehensive and withdrawn on the ward. He cried and whined and refused medication. When the parents were finally persuaded to let the boy's doctor discuss the disagnosis with him, his behavior changed radically. He became cheerful and relaxed and no longer refused his medications.

The mother of a 16-year-old patient spent all her energy during his illness "protecting" him from the truth. Twelve hours before he died, he asked her if he had leukemia. When she said yes, he told her, "Mother, I knew it all along." This patient "spent the last months of his life denied the emotional strength that his mother could have provided," Mr. Vernick points out.

Knowledge of his diagnosis is also a child's best defense against disastrous revelations from people outside the hospital. One 14-year-old boy was greeted on his return home by a friend who said, "You've got leukemia. You're supposed to be dead."

"Dead, hell," the boy snapped. "I'm here, ain't I?"

The Way It Was

LEECHING

As we were busy preparing the copy for this first issue of the newest addition to the nursing literature, it occurred to us to turn back to the past and to look into some of the early books on nursing published by the Saunders Company. Two of those we found were *Practical Points in Nursing,* by Emily A. M. Stoney, published in 1896 (this makes it one of the very first Saunders books), and *Modern Methods in Nursing,* by Georgiana J. Sanders (published in 1912). In both of these there were detailed and graphic descriptions of the process of leeching, designed to deprive the already ill patient of his life's blood. From them we learned some of the problems nurses had in those early days, for example:

In leeching, "care must be taken to apply the head and not the tail of the animal. The head is recognized by the three-cornered or Y-shaped mouth peculiar to the leech" (Sanders).

If the leech does not bite, "a drop of blood extracted from a pricked finger will generally cause the leech immediately to bite. Another very successful way is to put the leech in a very small wineglass or cup filled with water, in which it should remain for a few minutes; the edge of the wineglass is then held to the part we wish the leech to bite, and it will come up out of the water and generally take hold; should it move around, it can be guided to the right spot. As a leech is always hot and uncomfortable after being shut up in a box, it should be put into water (the glass or cup having a perforated paper cover) until we are ready to use it; being then in its natural element, it becomes cool and good-natured" (Stoney).

Or, "If the leech does not bite, he is usually hot, uncomfortable, and irritable, probably from having been kept out of water. He may be coaxed by smearing the part with milk, or by pricking the part until a drop of blood comes, or by gently stroking his back, but if still obstinate, it is quicker eventually to return him for a time to the water, and allow him to cool himself off in a dark place. A leech will frequently refuse to bite if the atmosphere of the room is heavy with tobacco or disinfectants, etc." (Sanders).

Then, "after the leech has taken hold, a piece of cotton should be slipped between it and the skin, because the movements of the leech give a very unplesant sensation to the patient, and tend to make some patients nervous. A leech generally holds from 1 to 2 teaspoonsful of blood, and when full it will drop off. If necessary to remove leeches after being on a certain length of time, a little salt sprinkled on their heads will make them drop off; they must not be pulled off, or they may leave their teeth in the wound and cause inflammation" (Stoney).

Disposing of leeches is done by "putting them into a very strong solution of salt and water or into dry salt, and covering the vessel tightly. The nurse must be sure they are dead before throwing them away" (Stoney).

INDEX

Acidosis, respiratory, in pulmonary emphysema, 42
Administrative responsibilities of pediatric nurse, 103–110
Ambulatory care in pediatrics, 76
Amniocentesis, 124
  nurse's role in, 126
Anxiety as reaction of nurse to ill child, 96
Arterial supply, reduced, conditions causing, 49

Bennett respirator, 143–152
  nursing responsibilities with, 147
  operation of, 146, 148
Blood dyscrasias, nursing care in, rationale of, 23–30
Blood incompatibilities, maternal-fetal, 123
  delivery in, 127
  nurse's role in, 125
Body surface area, determining drug dosage by, 112
Bronchitis, chronic, pathologic changes in, 39

Cardiac surgery, emotional stress in patient awaiting, 3–13
Cardiovascular disorders, in children, role of school nurse in, 31–38
Cardiovascular disorders, nursing problems in, 1–72
Cerebrovascular accident, definition, 63
  prevention, public health nurse's role in 64
  role of public health nurse, 63–72
  treatment, role of public health nurse, 66
  types, 63

Child, handicapped, discharged, role of public health nurse with, 153–162
  ill, nurse and, 73–162
    nurse's reaction to, 95–102
    medications for, physiological approach to, 111–120
Chloramphenicol, toxic effects in infant, 114
Clark's rule for pediatric drug dosage, 112
Congenital heart defects, in school children, 35
Connecticut Rheumatic Fever Prevention Program, 36
Consent, obtaining, for child patient, 104
Cor pulmonale, changes resulting from, 44

Digoxin, dosage for infant, 114
Dosages, drug, for children, 112
Drug administration, pediatric, physiological approach to, 111–120
Dyscrasias, blood, nursing care in, rationale of, 23–30

Embolus, with fractured hip, nurse's role in preventing, 59
Emotional stress in patient awaiting heart surgery, 3–13
Emphysema, pulmonary,
  complications and treatment, 42
    diagnostic and laboratory tests for, 41
  pathologic changes in, 39
  pulmonary circulation in, 39–46

Fetal medicine, role of nurse in, 121–129
Fetal transfusion, 125
  nurse's role in, 126

173

INDEX

Fetus, hazards to, 121
Fractured hip, prevention of circulatory complications in, 57–61

Gluteal muscles, use for intramuscular injections in children, 116

Handicapped child, discharged, role of public health nurse with, 153–162
Hartford Health Department project for Geriatric Medical Clinic, 66
Heart surgery, emotional stress in patient awaiting, 3–13
Hip, fractured, prevention of circulatory complications, 57–61
Hostility as reaction of nurse to ill child, 98
Hyperbaric oxygenation, definition, 131
nursing responsibility in planning for, 131–142

Injections, intramuscular, site for, in children, 116
Intermittent positive pressure breathing, 144
Intramuscular injections, site for, in children, 116
I.P.P.B., 144

Kanamycin, toxic effects of, 115

Leeching, 170
Leone, Lucile Petry, biography, 165
Leukemia, in children, 167

Maternal-fetal blood incompatibilities, 123
Medications, pediatric, physiological approach to, 111–120
Mothers, rooming-in for, meaning for nurse, 83–93. See also under *Rooming-in.*
Mount Sinai Hospital, hyperbaric oxygenation service in, 131–142

Newborn, drug dosage for, 114
Nurse, reaction of, to ill child, 95–102

Nursing and new pediatrics, 75–81
Nursing care in blood dyscrasias, rationale of, 23–30
Nursing care in hyperbaric oxygenation unit, 134
Nursing care in preventing circulatory complications in fractured hip, 57–61
Nursing care in vascular disease, 47–55
Nursing education, implications of new pediatrics, 80

Oxygenation, hyperbaric, nursing responsibilities in planning for, 131–142

Pediatric medications, physiological approach to, 111–120
Pediatric nurse, administrative responsibilities of, 103–110
reactions to ill child, 95–102
Pediatric rooming-in, meaning for nurse, 83–93
Pediatrics, new, nursing and, 75–81
social-behavioral orientation of, 75
Pericardium, sarcoma of, case study, 15–22
Peripheral vascular disease, etiology and symptoms, 47
nursing care in, 47–55
Polycythemia complicating pulmonary emphysema, 45
Positive pressure breathing, intermittent, 144
Premature, drug dosage for, 114
Preoperative period in heart surgery, 4
Public health nurse, preventive intervention by, with handicapped child, 156
role in cerebrovascular accident, 63–72
role with discharged handicapped child, 153–162
Pulmonary emphysema, pulmonary circulation in, 39–46
Pulmonary function, tests for, 41

Respiration, physiology of, 143
Respirator, Bennett, 143–152
nursing responsibilities with, 147
operation of 146, 148
Rh system incompatibilities, 124
Rheumatic fever, in school children, 34
prevention, 36
Rooming-in for mothers, desirability of, 85
meaning for nurse, 83–93

INDEX

Rooming-in for mothers (*Continued*)
  obstacles to, 92
  practical considerations, 91
  rationale of, 83
  role of mother in, 90
  role of nurse in, 88

Safety, responsibilities of pediatric nurse for, 108
Sarcoma of pericardium, case study, 15–22
School, role of professional nurse in, 31
School nurse, role of, in support of children with cardiovascular disorders, 31–38
Sciatic nerve damage due to intramuscular injections, 116

Stroke, role of public health nurse, 63–72. See also under *Cerebrovascular accident.*

Thrombosis, with fractured hip, nurse's role in preventing, 59
Thrombus formation, pathophysiology of, 58
Toxicity of drugs, for children, 115
Transfusion, intra-uterine, 125
  nurse's role in, 126

Vascular disease, nursing care in, 47–55
Venous flow, decreased, conditions causing, 49